ETHICAL DILEMMAS IN GENETICS AND GENETIC COUNSELING

Ethical Dilemmas in Genetics and Genetic Counseling

Principles through Case Scenarios

EDITED BY JANICE L. BERLINER

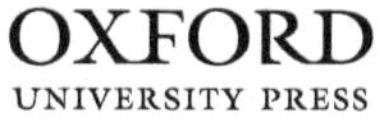

OXFORD
UNIVERSITY PRESS

Oxford University Press is a department of the University of Oxford. It furthers the University's objective of excellence in research, scholarship, and education by publishing worldwide.

Oxford New York
Auckland Cape Town Dar es Salaam Hong Kong Karachi
Kuala Lumpur Madrid Melbourne Mexico City Nairobi
New Delhi Shanghai Taipei Toronto

With offices in
Argentina Austria Brazil Chile Czech Republic France Greece
Guatemala Hungary Italy Japan Poland Portugal Singapore
South Korea Switzerland Thailand Turkey Ukraine Vietnam

Oxford is a registered trademark of Oxford University Press in the UK and certain other countries.

Published in the United States of America by
Oxford University Press
198 Madison Avenue, New York, NY 10016

Library of Congress Cataloging-in-Publication Data
Ethical dilemmas in genetics and genetic counseling : principles through case scenarios / edited by Janice L. Berliner.
p. ; cm.
ISBN 978-0-19-994489-7 (alk. paper)
I. Berliner, Janice L., editor.
[DNLM: 1. Genetic Counseling—ethics—Case Reports. 2. Ethical Analysis—Case Reports. 3. Genetic Testing—ethics—Case Reports. 4. Prenatal Diagnosis—ethics—Case Reports. QZ 50]
RB155
174.2′96042—dc23
2014019486

Contents

Contributors

Dawn C. Allain, MS, LGC
Division of Human Genetics, Department of Internal Medicine
The Ohio State University Wexner Medical Center
Columbus, OH

Rebecca R. Anderson, JD, MS, CGC
Department of Health Promotion, Social and Behavioral Health
College of Public Health
University of Nebraska Medical Center
Omaha, NE

Daragh Conrad, MS, CGC
Department of OB/GYN MFM
Comprehensive Fetal Care Center
Wake Forest Baptist Health
Winston-Salem, NC

Curtis R. Coughlin II, MS, MBe, CGC
Assistant Professor Pediatrics
Children's Hospital Colorado
University of Colorado School of Medicine
Aurora, CO

Sonja Eubanks Higgins, MS, CGC
Murrells Inlet, SC

Laura Hercher, MA, MS, CGC
Joan H. Marks Human Genetics Program
Sarah Lawrence College
Bronxville, NY

Kelly E. Ormond, MS, CGC
Department of Genetics and Stanford Center for Biomedical Ethics
Stanford University School of Medicine
Stanford, CA

Christy S. Stanley, MS, CGC
Department of OB/GYN MFM
Comprehensive Fetal Care Center
Wake Forest Baptist Health
Winston-Salem, NC

About the Editor

Janice L. Berliner, MS, CGC, has 25 years of experience in genetic counseling, primarily in cancer risk assessment. She provides education to health professionals and the community and also participates in research projects of the Clinical Genetics Service at Memorial Sloan Kettering Cancer Center. She has served on numerous committees as well as the Board of Directors of the National Society of Genetic Counselors and the American Board of Genetic Counseling.

ETHICAL DILEMMAS IN GENETICS AND GENETIC COUNSELING

1

Introduction to Clinical Ethics

REBECCA R. ANDERSON

The field of human genetics grows more complex and more vexing with each passing day. Scientists, clinicians, and patients struggle to understand floods of information, tantalizing and incomplete. They wrestle with ethical dilemmas posed by evolving technologies whose sequelae cannot be predicted. Meanwhile, policymakers are buffeted by constituencies clamoring for or against restrictions in research and practice.

Our guides through these thickets will be the members of the fictitious *Jones/Smith family*, depicted in Figure 1.1. With each chapter, we will examine some portion of their story in relation to an ethical issue posed by genetics in medical practice or research. Although the narrative builds from chapter to chapter, it is not necessary to read the book from beginning to end because each chapter stands on its own.

Chapter One offers an overview of medical ethics as it relates to human genetics. First, some basic definitions are in order.

The terms *moral* and *ethical* are used interchangeably in many contexts. Both terms refer to our sense of the good or the right, but not merely as matters of etiquette or social propriety. Rather, they are concerned with the most basic rules and commitments of human relationships and the management of divergent viewpoints and interests. Some people use the word *ethics* to denote the systematic analysis of what constitutes good or right behavior and *morals* to denote the underlying general principles.[i] Others advance different definitions.

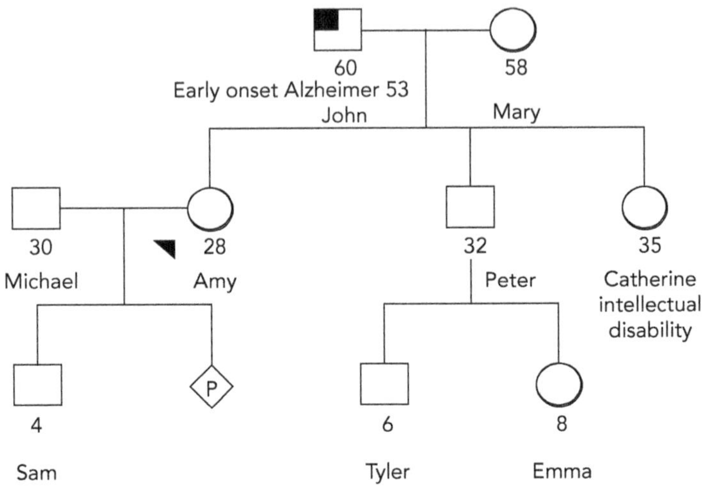

FIGURE 1.1 Amy, age 28, is the youngest daughter of John and Mary Jones. Amy is an accountant married to Michael Smith, a patent attorney. They have a healthy son, Sam, age 4, and Amy is pregnant. Amy's brother, Peter, is 32 and has two healthy children: Tyler, age 6 and Emma, age 8. Peter is an engineer and his wife, Joy, is a potter. Amy's oldest sibling, Catherine, is 35 and single. She has moderate intellectual disabilities secondary to complications of chicken pox. Since the age of 28 Catherine has lived in a group home and Amy has served as her legal guardian. Catherine's move from her parents' home was precipitated by early-onset Alzheimer in her father, John. A former banker, John began behaving erratically in his late 40s and was diagnosed with Alzheimer at 53. He tests positive for a dominant mutation in a presenilin gene, conferring a dramatically increased risk for early-onset dementia. Mary Jones continues to care for her husband at home but is finding this increasingly challenging as John's agitation and combativeness increase.

In this book we will use *moral* to refer to the convictions, conventions, and decisional processes guiding the good and the right in our nonprofessional lives. Moral convictions evolve from religious, philosophical, and cultural foundations (and possibly from genetic influences, but that's not a discussion for this text). Our legal system reflects widely shared moral convictions in both civil law (honoring one's promises in a contract, for example) and criminal law (punishing deliberate harm to another's person or property). Personal moral codes and principles often encompass thoughts, motives, and feelings as well as behaviors. Importantly, individuals choose their own sources of moral authority, and an authority persuasive to one person (e.g., a sacred text) may not be persuasive to another.

We will use *ethical* to refer to the convictions, conventions, and decisional processes guiding right behavior in professional life and in public policy. Although these definitions are somewhat arbitrary and carry significant overlap, the distinctions are useful, particularly when personal convictions of providers are in tension with professional expectations.[ii]

Although evolved from the same foundations as personal codes, professional codes of ethics, whether written or unwritten, tend to be more circumscribed. They reflect the custom and practice of skilled specialists who are pledged to use their training in the service of others. Ethical behavior for a professional may be defined by precedent as much as by adherence to principles and, as a rule, ethical precepts focus on behavior rather than on the internal processes of the actor.[iii]

In written form, professional codes, position statements, policies, guidelines, and practice parameters reflect peer consensus on appropriate behavior at the time of their adoption. Many such statements carry disclaimers, allowing individual providers to exercise their own judgment when departure from the norm is indicated. But professional behavior is not immune from outside influence. State licensure often governs entry into professional practice. Increasingly, state and federal statutes control key elements of the provider–patient relationship.[iv] Unless professional behavior meets a minimum *standard of care*, the professional may be civilly or criminally liable for failure to practice in a responsible manner.

The *standard of care* in the medical context typically measures the provider's acts (or failure to act) against those of a *reasonable and*

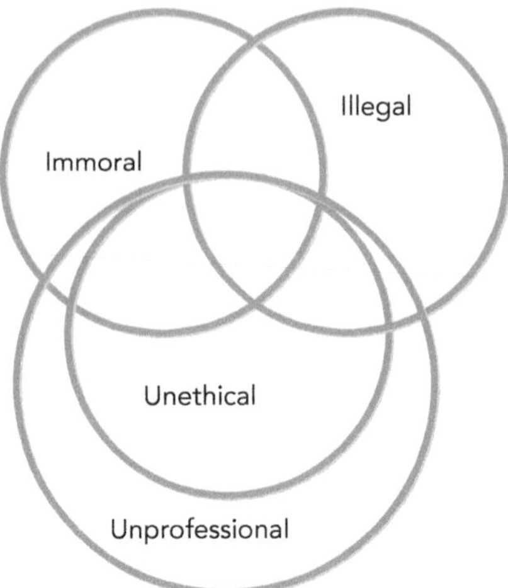

FIGURE 1.2 A single act may run afoul of only one of these categories, or may violate all four. If one has a consensual sexual relationship with someone to whom one is not married, one's behavior may be considered immoral but typically not unethical, unprofessional, or illegal. If one's intimate partner is a patient, one's behavior is both unethical and immoral. Such behavior violates regulatory but usually not criminal law: although one could lose one's license, one is not likely to go to jail. However, if that patient is 12 years of age, one has planted oneself in the middle of all four circles and can expect to do time.

prudent practitioner exercising *ordinary care and skill* under the *same or similar circumstances* in the *same or similar locality.*[v] State legislatures have adopted statutes defining the medical standard of care for their jurisdictions, and the courts apply those definitions when determining whether a provider has met the standard when the events in question took place (Figure 1.2).

Another ancient and central feature of professional practice (at least in law and medicine) is *fiduciary duty*. Because professionals possess knowledge and skills not commonly shared by lay people, their clients essentially are at their mercy. Clients may not even know the right questions to ask when they consult a professional and rarely are able to assess the accuracy or completeness of the information given them. Thus, as a matter of social contract, it is the duty of the professional to use his or her knowledge and skills for the benefit of the client—and not for the gain of others.

However, the boundaries of fiduciary duty may not end with the client or patient in the provider's care. For instance, if a patient is diagnosed with a serious and highly contagious disease, the provider may have a fiduciary duty to take action so that other people are not harmed.

Under what circumstances may a provider breach confidentiality to protect third parties? What should a provider do when a patient declines recommended therapy? What if a patient demands an intervention that is not medically appropriate or is against the convictions of the provider?

Such questions are the purview of *clinical* or *medical ethics.*

The rise of *medical ethics*[vi] as a discrete discipline was contemporaneous with the rise in scientific and technological capacity in the second half of the twentieth century. Unfortunately, human genetics provided some harrowing cautionary tales to the nascent field. In the early decades of the twentieth century, prominent US geneticists alleged they could identify inferior blood lines and advocated involuntary sterilization of the "unfit."[2,3,4] The notion was embraced and put into practice, with enabling legislation upheld by the US Supreme Court.[5] Following World War II and the exposure of the Nazi eugenics agenda,[vii] the scientific community no longer overtly promoted human eugenics—but some states continued to apply their sterilization laws until the 1970s.[2,3,4,viii]

Meanwhile, advances such as renal dialysis, artificial ventilation, and various "miracle drugs" forced providers and families to confront an unfamiliar problem in medicine: that of indefinitely forestalling death without restoring health. Prior to the advent of artificial respiration and nutrition, a patient who could not breathe, or could not manage food and fluids by mouth, died. With the advent of life-prolonging interventions came the question of when, and for whom, and for how long these interventions should be employed.

Into the public debate on these matters came news of scandalous abuses of research subjects at the hands of scientists at respected institutions. This prompted the adoption of new rules governing federally sponsored human research.[6] In addition, the federal government appointed a commission to identify salient ethical principles and recommend appropriate ways to honor them. The resulting 1978 *Belmont Report*[7] identified *respect for persons, beneficence,* and *justice* as the central ethical themes in human subjects research. This triad (often denoted *autonomy, beneficence/nonmaleficence, and justice*) quickly was adopted for medical ethics discourse in general.

Autonomy is analogous to the legal principle of self-determination. It presumes that adults of sound mind should be free to govern their own affairs, as long as they don't infringe on the rights of others. A substitute decision maker exercises this right on behalf of a minor[ix] or incapacitated person.

Providers are obligated to facilitate the exercise of self-determination by assessing decisional capacity, guarding against coercion or undue influence, eliciting the patient's goals and values, providing full and timely information about a patient's medical status and treatment options, offering professional advice, and honoring the patient's considered decisions. Providers are *not* obligated to perform medically inappropriate interventions, even if patients earnestly desire them. Autonomy is not limitless.

Beneficence means doing good. *Nonmaleficence* means avoiding harm. Ordinarily the law does not require that we come to the aid of strangers—but we are expected not to hurt them. And the law does require that we act to benefit others under certain circumstances. Relationships create duties. Parents have enforceable duties to minor children; healthcare providers have duties to their patients; lawyers have duties to their clients and to the courts.

Providers honor the principle of beneficence by offering appropriate interventions, discussing options thoroughly, and performing their tasks skillfully. They honor the principle of nonmaleficence by declining to offer or perform interventions if there is no reasonable chance of success or if the likely burdens substantially outweigh the potential benefits. They avoid harm by inviting patients to consider long-term as well as short-term consequences of their choices and by attending to the psychosocial dimensions of patient care.

Justice asks that burdens and benefits be distributed fairly, and that insofar as possible people are "made whole," in essence restored to their former status after they have suffered harm. In the legal realm, justice means more than punishing the guilty and absolving the innocent. It implies an orderly system in which well-considered laws are appropriately enforced and consistently applied. In the medical realm justice is more frequently invoked at the policy level than at the bedside, but in both settings the allocation of scarce resources often is the focus.

At the bedside, providers honor the principle of justice by declining (except in rare instances such as voluntary donation of organs or tissues) to harm one person in order to help another. They base treatment choices on medical considerations rather than on race, age, disability, socioeconomic status, or other characteristics not relevant to the safety and efficacy of an intervention, particularly when demand exceeds supply. They open research studies to all qualifying patients and assure that research design protects the interests of subjects, being especially mindful of coercion or misapprehension of the research endeavor.

In the public policy realm, different theories of justice and fairness may produce markedly different recommendations about how our medical system should be managed. A person who advocates "the greatest good for the greatest number" is more likely to endorse mandatory vaccinations than a person for whom individual liberty is the primary value. A person who believes that hard work and self-sufficiency are essential to human integrity may not embrace tax-supported medical services for the disadvantaged.

In our pluralistic society, policy discussions must elicit and give due consideration to a wide range of values and priorities. Genetic advances bring into close focus some of our most divisive topics.

Many touch on "ultimate questions," such as what it means to be human, what duties we owe to one another as persons, and how we allocate power and responsibility, particularly in our reproductive lives. Some of these questions simply are beyond the scope of science. No empirical study will tell us what constitutes personhood or when during the course of development a person comes into being. There are (or used to be) legal answers to that question. In common law[x] a child born alive was a person and thus an heir; a child miscarried or stillborn was not.[8,9,xi] Although the same logic banned recovery for fetal death following an attack on a pregnant woman, in recent years some states have extended civil and criminal liability to these events.[9]

Jewish theology mirrors the common law understanding that a fetus is not a person until born alive. Until the first breath is taken, the fetus has lesser claims upon the community of faith. A stillborn, while treated with respect, is not accorded full mourning rites. Until the moment of birth, the mother's health takes priority over that of the fetus. Indeed, if a mother's life is threatened by a continuing pregnancy, Jewish law requires that she be delivered regardless of the consequences to the fetus.[10,11]

In contrast, contemporary Roman Catholic and Orthodox Christian theologies identify the moment of conception as the beginning of personhood.[12,13,xii] Accordingly, while a woman may be permitted to end a pregnancy if her life is threatened, she is revered as a martyr if she refuses to do so.[12,13,14,xiii]

People who do not subscribe to a faith tradition likewise differ in their assessments of when personhood begins and ends, and what it means. Particularly when considering liminal stages of existence—for example in vitro pre-embryos, persistent vegetative state—arguments about the duties we owe and the acts in which we may engage necessarily are made on moral and ethical rather than scientific grounds. The same may be said of debates about altering the genetic code of living organisms, whether by traditional or novel means. Science can inform but not settle our questions about limits. If we are serious as a society about preserving freedom of—and from—religion, how do we accommodate such divergent beliefs? And what are the limits of our accommodation?

Careful ethical analysis for public policy purposes requires that we learn as much as possible about the biological systems in question and then acknowledge that our current understanding may be wrong. We then must evaluate, as objectively as we can, the range of outcomes flowing from various choices for the individual as well as for society. We must ask time-honored questions: "What would happen if everyone chose this?" "Does this treat people as mere means to an end?" "Does the risk-to-benefit ratio justify the intervention?" "Will some members of society (especially the vulnerable) be disproportionately harmed?" "If we spend our resources here, what else will go unfunded?" In many respects we are asking how the proposed activity squares with our collective notions of liberty, goodness, virtue, justice...and only by asking the questions can we uncover the shapes of those collective notions, because they take different shapes in different circumstances.

Perhaps we can best support the moral agency of individuals by maximizing choice within generally accepted boundaries. The role of law and professional ethics is to establish those boundaries. The role of the provider is to describe the territory within those boundaries by providing full and fair information about all legal, medically appropriate options so that the patient can exercise his or her own judgment about how to proceed. Fiduciary duty requires no less. Clinical genetics embraces this tradition in nondirective counseling. Its purpose is not to avoid making recommendations (particularly with regard to medical management) but to facilitate patient-centered choices.

When a patient is facing an emotionally freighted choice, a provider may worry that even the mention of a controversial option will be taken by the patient as a recommendation or endorsement. In these situations it may be helpful to say, "It is within your rights to [end the pregnancy] [decline prenatal testing] [stop the breathing machine]. Is that something you might want to consider?" This signals the legal availability of a medically acceptable option, and if the patient wishes to learn more, he or she generally says so. If not, the provider has satisfied the duty to make the patient aware of the choice without undermining trust.

Ultimately, fiduciary responsibility requires that providers acknowledge that their own moral convictions cannot trump those of their patients. A provider who is morally opposed to a legal and medically appropriate intervention need not participate in the intervention[xiv] but must make sure the patient is aware of its availability and must give the patient sufficient information to make a timely, informed choice. If a provider is unable to do so, then the provider has an ethical obligation to inform the patient of his or her practice limitations and offer to refer the patient to a neutral third party able to assist the patient in securing the information elsewhere.

Clinically, ethical dilemmas often arise when there is disagreement among family members or care providers about the proper course of treatment. But that alone rarely precipitates an ethics consultation.[15,xv] Usually at least one other factor is present: questions about the decisional capacity of the patient or the good faith of the substitute decision maker; uncertainty about the goals of intervention and whether those goals can be achieved; questions about proportionality (burden vs. benefit, or use of an extremely costly or scarce resource in the face of a low probability of success); questions about quality of life; questions about law, beliefs, family dynamics, and so forth.

There are many approaches to ethical analysis—virtue ethics, narrative ethics, feminist ethics, ethics of care, religious ethics, deontology or principles-based ethics, utilitarianism, communitarianism —each emphasizing slightly different values but all intending to seek balance and a just result. Few ethicists dealing with a clinical problem are seeking "the" right answer—rather, the goal in most cases is to avoid obviously wrong answers and come to a consensus on one of several right answers.

One particularly user-friendly assessment strategy has been advanced by ethicists Albert Jonsen (philosopher), Mark Siegler (physician), and William Winslade (attorney). Table 1.1 depicts the central themes of their work.

Use of this chart as a template makes ethical analysis less daunting to families and providers. It is amenable to prenatal, preconception, and predictive testing issues as well as more traditional clinical questions.

Analysis begins with the top two boxes. The authors note that if the medical issues and options are well understood and a patient with decisional capacity makes an informed, considered choice, then that is the end of the matter: the patient's preferences prevail. But if assessment of the top boxes does not cover all of the salient issues, the lower boxes come into play. Assessing a patient's prospective quality of life is never easy, but the questions posed can help families and providers examine these matters more systematically. The final box, contextual features, is of particular importance because it brings to the foreground considerations that may otherwise be unvoiced, such as the impact of a decision upon other family members.

Once the grid has been completed and the parties have come to a fuller understanding of the landscape, it may be useful to reassess the goals of care, based upon what is represented. It may be useful to identify the areas of agreement and work into the areas of disagreement. Since ethical dilemmas at the bedside often focus on whether to undertake a particular medical intervention for a gravely ill individual, it is often helpful to remind participants that regardless of the decision made, medical care and comfort measures will continue. We never "discontinue care" even though we may decide against a procedure.

In clinical genetics, a gravely ill individual is not often at the center of the ethical dilemma. Ethical issues are more likely to involve reproductive technologies and the inherent tensions in the maternal–fetal dyad, management of "incidental" or "secondary" genetic information in ever-expanding test panels, predictive testing,

TABLE 1.1 The Four Topics Chart

Medical Indications	Patient Preferences
The Principles of Beneficence and Nonmaleficence What is the patient's medical problem? Is the problem acute? Chronic? Critical? Reversible? Emergent? Terminal? What are the goals of treatment? In what circumstances are medical treatments not indicated? What are the probabilities of success of various treatment options? In sum, how can this patient be benefited by medical and nursing care, and how can harm be avoided?	*The Principle of Respect for Autonomy* Has the patient been informed of benefits and risks, understood this information, and given consent? Is the patient mentally capable and legally competent, and is there evidence of incapacity? If mentally capable, what preferences about treatment is the patient stating? If incapacitated, has the patient expressed prior preferences? Who is the appropriate surrogate to make decisions for the incapacitated patient? Is the patient unwilling or unable to cooperate with medical treatment? If so, why?
Quality of Life	**Contextual Features**
The Principles of Beneficence and Nonmaleficence and Respect for Autonomy What are the prospects, with or without treatment, for a return to normal life, and what physical, mental, and social deficits might the patient experience even if treatment succeeds?	*The Principles of Justice and Fairness* Are there professional, interprofessional, or business interests that might create conflicts of interest in the clinical treatment of patients? Are there parties other than clinicians and patients, such as family members, who have an interest in clinical decisions?

(*continued*)

TABLE 1.1 Continued

On what grounds can anyone judge that some quality of life would be undesirable for a patient who cannot make or express such a judgment? Are there biases that might prejudice the provider's evaluation of the patient's quality of life? Do quality-of-life assessments raise any questions regarding changes in treatment plans, such as forgoing life-sustaining treatment? What is the legal and ethical status of suicide?	What are the limits imposed on patient confidentiality by the legitimate interests of third parties? Are there financial factors that create conflicts of interest in clinical decisions? Are there problems of allocation of scarce health resources that might affect clinical decisions? Are there religious issues that might influence clinical decisions? What are the legal issues that might affect clinical decisions? Are there considerations of clinical research and education that might affect clinical decisions? Are there issues of public health and safety that affect clinical decisions? Are there conflicts of interest within institutions and organizations (e.g., hospitals) that may affect clinical decisions and patient welfare?

Jonsen, A.R., Siegler, M. and Winslade W.J. *Clinical Ethics: A Practical Approach to Ethical Decisions in Clinical Medicine*. 7th ed. New York, NY: McGraw-Hill; 2010.

experimental use of residual specimens, and the like. Apart from the prenatal setting, decisions are rarely urgent. But choices made by one family member may have profound consequences for other family members, who may not be parties to the discussion. Attention should be paid to the wider ramifications of potential choices.

A careful ethical analysis is likely to exclude some options because they are not medically appropriate, and it may exclude other options because they are not consonant with family goals and values. Some alternatives may be seen as resulting in an unacceptably poor quality of life. Ethical discourse may also lead to the realization that a different person should act as the substitute decision maker for a patient who lacks capacity. But ultimately, within the acceptable alternatives, a decision must be made—whether it be to undertake an intervention or decline it.

At this juncture it may be useful to ask, "What is the most loving thing to do?" A response to this query necessarily flows from the core values of the family. Answering it requires contemplation of the lived experience of each alternative and invites reflection about how one will look back on the decision in the future. In the long run, a family choosing its path on this basis is more likely to be at peace.

NOTES

i. *Ethics*, the philosophical study of morality. The word is also commonly used interchangeably with "morality" to mean the subject matter of this study, and sometimes it is used more narrowly to mean the moral principles of a particular tradition, group, or individual.[1]

ii. *Professionalism* embraces not only ethical behavior but also etiquette and custom, for example civility, neatness in appearance, and so forth.

iii. *Professional ethics* is a term designating one or more of (1) the justified moral values that should govern the work of professionals; (2) the moral values that actually do guide groups of professionals, whether those values are identified as (a) principles in codes of ethics promulgated by professional societies or (b) actual beliefs and conduct of professionals; and (3) the study of professional ethics in the preceding senses. Professions are defined by advanced expertise, social organizations, society-granted monopolies over services, and especially by shared commitments to promote a distinctive public good such as health (medicine), justice (law), or learning (education). These shared commitments imply special duties to make services available, maintain confidentiality, secure informed consent for services, and be loyal to clients, employers, and others with whom one has fiduciary relationships.[1]

iv. In the United States, confidentiality is governed by federal (HIPAA) as well as state statutes. Several states have passed laws and regulations mandating particular content in informed consent documents relating to genetic testing. Statutes governing prenatal diagnosis and pregnancy interruption are subject to frequent change, and with the passage of the Partial Birth Abortion Ban Act of 2003 (18 U.S.C. 1531 *et seq*) Congress has signaled its intention to take a more active role in this domain.

v. See, for example, Neb. Rev. Stat. 44-2810 (malpractice or professional negligence, defined): Malpractice or professional negligence shall mean that, in rendering professional services, a health care provider has failed to use the ordinary and reasonable care, skill, and knowledge ordinarily possessed and used under like circumstances by members of his profession engaged in a similar practice in his or in similar localities. In determining what constitutes reasonable and ordinary care, skill, and diligence on the part of a health care provider in a particular community, the test shall be that which health care providers, in the same community or in similar communities and engaged in the same or similar lines of work, would ordinarily exercise and devote to the benefit of their patients under like circumstances.

vi. The term *clinical ethics* typically refers to the analysis and resolution of actual patient-provider issues. The term *medical ethics* includes clinical and research ethics as well as public policy issues related to human health. The term *bioethics* describes a broad discipline exploring the ramifications of scientific advances and new technologies across species and environments. Writings in this field often adopt a wider, more speculative view but also deal with traditional medical ethics.

vii. The American eugenics movement allegedly served as a template for the Nazi eugenics movement.[2,3,4] Other WWII outrages involving physicians complicit in torture and forced experimentation led to the promulgation in 1947 of the *Nuremberg Code*[17] and in 1948 of the *Declaration of Geneva*. The former established principles for human subjects research; the latter articulated basic ethical obligations of physicians. When further research scandals were brought to light in the United States, these two documents (with subsequent revisions) became the foundation for the *Common Rule*[6] adopted by Congress in 1975 to govern the conduct of federally funded research. Among other things this law requires that

Institutional Review Boards (IRBs) review and approve human subjects research to assure that informed consent is obtained, risks and benefits are carefully considered, and scientific merit is demonstrated. Research funded through other sources is not subject to the Common Rule, but many privately funded investigators comply with it because most scientific journals require evidence of IRB approval prior to publication.

viii. The Cold Spring Harbor Laboratory DNA Learning Center provides fine coverage of the American eugenics movement.[2,3,4]

ix. Although parents have considerable discretion in directing the medical care of their minor children, the state also has an interest in preserving the lives and future decision-making authority of minors. Hence, the state may intervene to require some medical interventions and prohibit others.

x. Common law is the law articulated over the centuries through court decisions. Statutory law is enacted by legislatures. Many statutes are essentially restatements of common law, but when a statute codifies a principle of common law, the language of the statute takes priority over other interpretations.

xi. Infants Existence Inchoate and Conditional – the existence of a child *en ventre sa mere* is inchoate and conditional, and confers no right of property unless the infant be born alive after such a period of foetal existence that its continuance in life may reasonably be expected; and if it is born dead, or in such an early stage of pregnancy as to be incapable of living, it is to be considered as if it had never been born or conceived. Consequently a person claiming property through such a child is bound to establish the fact that it was born alive.[8]

xii. Interestingly, until recently, no committal or mourning rituals were observed for pregnancy loss in these traditions, although some Orthodox liturgical prayers asked forgiveness for the "intentional or unintentional sins" of the mother that caused the fetal demise.[12]

xiii. Orthodox Church in America: In those increasingly rare cases where a medical choice must be made between the life of the mother and that of her unborn child, it is morally permissible to favor the mother. This is not because she is a full "person" whereas the fetus is merely "potential life," for both are equally human. It is rather because of the mother's place and responsibility within the family, where her nurturing and loving presence directly affects the lives of her husband and other children.

Nevertheless, a mother who willingly surrenders her own life in favor of her infant performs the profoundest act of Christian charity. "Greater love has no one than this," Jesus declares, "than that he lay down his life for his friend."[12] Roman Catholic Church: Abortion (that is, the directly intended termination of pregnancy before viability or the directly intended destruction of a viable fetus) is never permitted. Every procedure whose sole immediate effect is the termination of pregnancy before viability is an abortion, which, in its moral context, includes the interval between conception and implantation of the embryo. [...] Operations, treatments, and medications that have as their direct purpose the cure of a proportionately serious pathological condition of a pregnant woman are permitted when they cannot be safely postponed until the unborn child is viable, even if they will result in the death of the unborn child. In the case of an extrauterine pregnancy, no intervention is morally licit which constitutes a direct abortion. For a proportionate reason, labor may be induced after the fetus is viable.[14]

xiv. On rare occasion a provider may be obliged to engage in an intervention he or she considers morally objectionable, because failing to do so would result in patient abandonment. Typically, employers outline in their policies and procedures the processes available to opt out of a practice to which the provider is morally opposed.

xv. All hospitals are required by JCAHO, the Joint Commission for Accreditation of Healthcare Organizations, to have a system in place to resolve ethical questions in health care. The system need not take the form of an ethics consultation service, but many hospitals (particularly academic hospitals) offer a formal ethics consultation mechanism. Independent providers may be able to consult with ethicists at their state universities or with their professional organizations but will not be able to share privileged information without patient permission. For a discussion of standards for ethics consultation, see *Health ethics consultation: an update on core competencies and emerging standards* from the American Society for Bioethics and Humanities' core competencies update task force.[15]

REFERENCES

1. Audi, R., ed. (1999). *The Cambridge Dictionary of Philosophy*, 2nd edition. Cambridge University Press.

2. http://blogs.dnalc.org/category/sitetopics/eugenicsarchive/. Accessed April 28, 2014.
3. http://www.eugenicsarchive.org/eugenics/list2.pl. Accessed April 28, 2014.
4. http://www.dnai.org/e/index.html. Accessed July 20, 2013.
5. Buck v. Bell, 274 U.S. 200, 1927.
6. http://www.hhs.gov/ohrp/humansubjects/guidance/45cfr46.html. Accessed July 20, 2013.
7. http://www.hhs.gov/ohrp/humansubjects/guidance/belmont.html. Accessed July 20, 2013.
8. Garland, D.S., McGehee, L.P., eds. *The American and English Encyclopedia of Law*, 2nd edition. Long Island, NY, London: Edward Thompson Co. (1900) v. XVI p. 260. Hathi Trust Digital Library. http://babel.hathitrust.org/cgi/pt?id=nyp.33433008086302;view=1up;seq=272. Accessed August 6, 2013.
9. National Conference of State Legislatures. Fetal Homicide Laws, updated February 2013. http://www.ncsl.org/issues-research/health/fetal-homicide-state-laws.aspx. Accessed April 28, 2014.
10. Dorff, E. (1999). *Matters of Life and Death: Modern Jewish Medical Ethics*. pp. 14–37, 128–133. Philadelphia and Jerusalem: The Jewish Publication Society.
11. Anderson, R. (2002). *Religions Traditions and Prenatal Genetic Counseling*. Omaha, NE: Munroe Meyer Institute, University of Nebraska Medical Center.
12. Breck, J. (1998). *The Sacred Gift of Life: Orthodox Christianity and Bioethics*. Crestwood, NY: St. Vladimir's Seminary Press.
13. Catholic News Agency. "Emotional farewell for young Italian mother who died for unborn child." http://www.catholicnewsagency.com/news/emotional-goodbye-for-young-italian-mother-who-died-for-unborn-child/. Accessed July 20, 2013.
14. United States Conference of Catholic Bishops. (2009). *Ethical and Religious Directives for Catholic Health Care Services*. 5th edition. Available at: http://www.usccb.org/issues-and-action/human-life-and-dignity/health-care/upload/Ethical-Religious-Directives-Catholic-Health-Care-Services-fifth-edition-2009.pdf. Accessed July 20, 2013.
15. Tarzian, A.J., ASBH Core Competencies Update Task Force 1. (2013). Health ethics consultation: an update on core competencies

and emerging standards from the American Society for Bioethics and Humanities' core competencies update task force. *American Journal of Bioethics*. 13(2):3–13.
16. Jonsen, A.R., Siegler, M., Winslade, W.J. (2010). *Clinical Ethics: A Practical Approach to Ethical Decisions in Clinical Medicine*. 7th edition. New York: McGraw-Hill.
17. US Department of Health and Human Services. *The Nuremberg Code*. Available at: http://www.hhs.gov/ohrp/archive/nurcode.html. Accessed March 1, 2013.

2

The (micro) Array of Options for Prenatal Testing

DARAGH CONRAD AND CHRISTY S. STANLEY

At the heart of the genetic counselor's role in a prenatal setting is the concept of nondirective counseling. This tenet contrasts with the traditional physician role in medicine where the provider acts as the expert. This is also in contrast with most patients' typical experiences with other healthcare providers. Nondirectiveness allows for patient autonomy in reproduction. Historically, it was thought that nondirectiveness was crucial in prenatal genetic counseling solely to avoid the perception of eugenics. However, it is important to see that the highly personal nature of prenatal genetic counseling, in that it involves family planning and reproductive choices, requires a higher level of caution for reasons other than simply the avoidance of eugenics. A patient's personal value system and life views come into play in ways that they do not in other areas of medicine or even in other areas of prenatal care. Many prenatal counselors are still pressed by their patients for a directive approach. In all but rare instances, there is not a "right" answer. There is the answer that is right for the family or that seems "most right" at the time when the decision needs to be made. And this is true whether a family is deciding whether to have a screening test, to decline the option for an invasive test that carries a risk of pregnancy loss, or to determine if they will choose to continue a pregnancy. In none of these situations is there a "right" path to choose. There is only the path that is right for *that* patient at *that* time.

Parents attempt to act or may be conditioned to behave in a way that protects their children. This is a primordial instinct in many ways. This need includes protecting children from disease. Even regarding this basic tenet, parents behave differently. For example, some parents will choose to vaccinate their children to protect them from disease. Others feel that they are providing better protection by not subjecting their children to immunizations. In each case, the parents are doing what they believe to be "right." This need to watch over offspring does not begin when they are born; it starts when the child is in the womb. Parents want to protect their unborn children from disease and other disorders. While the common question in pregnancy is "do you want a boy or a girl?" and many parents have an expressed or unexpressed preference, most will answer, "as long as it's healthy, we will be happy." There is an unquestionable and innate desire to have a healthy pregnancy and healthy child(ren). While so many factors in pregnancy are beyond parental control, parents desire to manage those things that can be altered. This may manifest as eating better during pregnancy, taking prenatal vitamins, exercising, or eliminating alcohol or smoking, but it can also be seen in how one approaches prenatal testing and screening.

The genetics revolution has created a flood of information, and popular media together with the Internet has spread the message that there are more opportunities to test during pregnancy. Importantly, none of these tests can change the "genetics" of the baby. That information is set at conception, or really prior to conception at the time of maturation of the egg and sperm cells. Technology simply allows parents greater insight into what those genetics are or will be. Even so, the information does not necessarily identify how that genetic material will be manifested in a baby. However, the implication is that not taking advantage of available technology means one is missing out or shortchanging oneself or the unborn baby.

New technologies are replacing the more traditional testing and screening options. With ever greater use, costs are coming down and availability is increasing. But this opportunity also creates new, clinically relevant, ethical issues.

Prenatal testing and screening, while having similarities, are different in their origins and their roles in prenatal care. Prenatal *testing* is considered to be diagnostic. It identifies the presence or absence of one or more specific conditions in a fetus, with the degree of accuracy of the test dependent upon that test's particular sensitivity and specificity. In order to be diagnostic, a specific fetal sample is necessary. Prenatal *screening,* on the other hand, is designed either to adjust the likelihood that a fetus has a particular condition (or one of several conditions) or to screen the pregnant population for specific disorders. Some conditions are included within a screening paradigm because of their frequency in the general population or because there is a benefit to the baby at birth or improved outcome with prenatal diagnosis. There remains a pervasive thought that screening and testing are designed to eradicate from the world a particular genetic condition (reminiscent of eugenics), while in reality prenatal diagnosis and screening are used to improve the outcome for all babies, with and without prenatally diagnosed conditions. It is well documented that knowing ahead of time about a fetal anomaly, such as a neural tube defect (NTD), improves the outcome for that baby. While some families may deliver at a tertiary care center simply because of geography, others would not typically do so. Prenatal diagnosis of health conditions requiring early or immediate intervention allows for changes in delivery timing and location to allow for appropriate and intensive care.

While prenatal testing historically involves an invasive test, either amniocentesis or chorionic villi sampling (CVS), prenatal screening typically is a less invasive process utilizing a maternal blood sample or fetal ultrasound. Unlike diagnostic testing, screening is unlikely to pose a risk to the mother or the developing baby. This benefit of screening often makes it a more desirable option, and the acceptance of some form of prenatal screening is generally high. However, screening is not without its own set of consequences. Most parents expect the screening process to result in a reduction of risk such that they can sit back, relax, and enjoy the remainder of their pregnancy, and for most it follows this planned path. Unfortunately, for a small percentage of parents the results of the screening are not what they expected. The selected screening test results in an increased or intermediate risk leading them down a very different path of additional screening or toward the option of testing. One must consider both potential outcomes when considering whether to proceed with screening. This may or may not be a path on which a parent wants to start. For that reason, even a test without a risk to mom or developing baby still must be evaluated and counseled about, not just ordered like a complete blood count (CBC).

Prenatal testing and termination of pregnancy have been (rightly or wrongly) linked together. This does not mean to imply that one leads to the other or that the only reason to engage in testing or screening is to make a pregnancy-related decision. However, one participates in prenatal testing or screening to learn more about a pregnancy. What one elects to do with the information learned from that endeavor will vary based upon the results, the perception of the disease burden, the person's own beliefs, and a multitude of other factors. To believe that one can discuss one without thought of the other is simply wrong, and to provide complete counseling requires discussion of both.

Alpha-fetoprotein (AFP) was discovered in cancer research during the 1960s. In the 1970s the idea of screening for (NTDs) by measuring AFP in maternal serum was proposed. It was because of these screening programs that ultimately the observation was made that serum AFP concentrations were lower in pregnancies with Down syndrome. This evolved into screening programs for Down syndrome and NTDs. As time passed and knowledge expanded, so did screening programs. What began as single-marker screening evolved into the double screen with the addition of human chorionic gonadotropin (AFP/hCG), then the triple screen after the addition of unconjugated estriol (AFP/hCG/uE3), and finally the quad screen with the addition of diametric inhibin A (DIA). This screening was limited in its scope as it adjusted the risk for a well-defined, well-understood set of conditions (NTDs, Down syndrome, and Trisomy 18). Regardless of the markers used in the maternal serum screening, it was a simple one-step test that a woman could accept or decline early in the second trimester of pregnancy.

As ultrasound technology improved, second trimester ultrasound became more reliable in the detection of fetal anomalies and in the ability, through the presence or absence of soft markers, to modify an a priori risk for specific chromosome conditions. With the advent of first trimester ultrasound for measurement of fetal nuchal translucency, the era of first trimester screening began. With it came the ability to identify fetuses at risk for chromosome conditions in the first trimester of pregnancy. As this screening expanded, it was also recognized that an increased fetal nuchal translucency (NT) was associated with fetal cardiac defects and numerous other genetic conditions in a developing fetus. We had moved from screening for a small, clearly defined set of conditions to what was becoming an endless list of possible conditions with an unclear detection rate. NT-based screening was, on the surface, screening for a small set of defined chromosome conditions, but in reality could open up a Pandora's Box of information which the patient may not have asked for or wanted.

Amniocentesis, in many respects, launched the era of prenatal diagnosis for genetic disorders and congenital anomalies. The first report of evaluation of the fetal chromosome constitution occurred in 1966. Soon after, there were reports of diagnoses of chromosome conditions and then metabolic conditions identified in amniotic fluid cells. Amniocentesis and CVS were traditionally used in "high-risk" pregnancies to confirm or exclude a specific condition for which the fetus had been determined to have an increased risk. This assessment of risk was based on maternal condition (age or medical condition), family history, or prior screening test. As prenatal screening existed for only a very few specific genetic conditions, prenatal diagnostic testing was only provided for a limited number of clearly defined conditions.

The launch of new testing has changed all of that, particularly when it is used in the prenatal realm. Fetal cells, once they have been obtained from invasive testing, can be used in many different ways to identify hundreds of other conditions. In other circumstances invasive testing is not necessary to acquire fetal DNA, increasing the complexity of informing parents of their available options. Whole genome sequencing (sequencing analysis of an individual's entire genome) and whole exome sequencing (sequencing analysis of an individual's exons), as well as microarray analysis (analysis for deletions or duplications of particular regions of the genome), significantly increase the chance of identifying a relevant disorder. However, they exponentially increase the chance that an unwanted or unclear finding may be revealed.

Noninvasive Prenatal Testing

Since the 1970s, researchers have been interested in obtaining fetal DNA from maternal circulation for use in the detection of fetal aneuploidy. Initial efforts were directed at isolation of intact fetal cells, including fetal lymphocytes and isolated nucleated red blood cells (RBCs). Bianchi et al first detected a 47, XY+21 fetal karyotype in maternal peripheral blood utilizing FISH techniques in 1992.[1] This method had various limitations, including low concentration of intact fetal cells in maternal circulation and persistence of intact fetal cells from prior pregnancies (intact fetal cells can remain in maternal circulation for years). Investigators then focused on analysis of circulating cell-free fetal DNA (cffDNA). This inspiration came from reports of tumor DNA being detected in the plasma or serum of patients with cancer. YM Dennis Lo and colleagues were the first to report detection of circulating cffDNA in maternal blood.[2] They included analysis of 43 maternal samples

(30 from mothers with male fetuses and 13 from mothers with female fetuses) including a plasma, serum, and nucleated RBC sample from each. Results showed that Y sequences were detected in 24 of 30 (80%) of the maternal plasma samples, 21 of 30 (70%) of the serum samples, and 5 of 30 (17%) of the nucleated RBC samples. None of the 13 samples of mothers with female fetuses had positive results. Lo concluded, "Our finding of circulating fetal DNA in maternal plasma may have implications for non-invasive prenatal diagnosis, and for improving our understanding of the fetomaternal relationship." This, in many ways, began a paradigm shift in the practice of prenatal screening/diagnosis.

Cell-free fetal DNA can be detected by the 7th week of gestation, with relatively stable amounts found between 10 and 20 weeks gestation. It coexists with a large background of maternal cell-free DNA; however, it is rapidly removed from maternal circulation within hours of delivery. It is, therefore, a genetic snapshot of the current pregnancy without influence from prior pregnancies. This technology was initially directed toward detection of unique paternally inherited traits, which would be exclusive to the fetus and distinguishable from the maternal DNA sequences. This included fetal sex determination and fetal rhesus D (RhD) status determination. More recent research has focused on screening for fetal aneuploidy.

Identification of fetal aneuploidy is more complicated than determination of fetal sex or RhD status, because there are no unique fetal gene sequences to be detected. The arrival of mass parallel shotgun sequencing enhanced the progress in the detection of fetal aneuploidy from cell-free fetal DNA in maternal plasma. In 2008, the first studies documented the detection of fetal aneuploidy utilizing cffDNA isolated from maternal plasma by mapping and aligning short sequence tags to a reference human genome. This was followed by counting and bioinformatics analyses. Since 2011, more than 20 large-scale studies involving noninvasive prenatal testing (NIPT) of trisomy 21, trisomy 13, and trisomy 18 have been published. The majority of the studies have focused on "high risk" patients with singleton pregnancies. The term *high risk* generally is used to refer to those patients with a risk for fetal aneuploidy that is greater than or equal to the risk for pregnancy loss associated with diagnostic testing, (e.g., advanced maternal age, abnormal maternal serum biochemical or combined screening result, family history concerns, or anomalies or soft markers for fetal aneuploidy detected by ultrasound). Studies have found near-perfect rates of detection for Down syndrome (including, but not distinguishing between, trisomy 21, translocation Down syndrome, and mosaic Down syndrome).[3,4,5,6,7] The false-positive rates (FPR) are estimated to be less than 1% and in most studies are approximately 0.1%. The detection rate for trisomy 18 and 13 has been found to be slightly lower, with an equally low FPR.[4,5,6] The lower detection rate for trisomy 13 is thought to be due to the guanine and cytosine content of the DNA and/or the rarity of the condition. Analysis of the X chromosome for sex chromosome aneuploidy has been more recently investigated and is now also commercially available.[8,9] The detection rate varies depending on the study but is comparable to the detection rates for the other chromosomes studied. Multiple commercial laboratories offer NIPT, using a variety of methodologies including mass parallel shotgun sequencing, targeted sequencing, and single nucleotide polymorphism (genotyping). The methodology influences the detection rate, false-positive rate, and cost of the testing.

Both twin and low-risk studies have been published and the data is promising, suggesting that this testing methodology will perform well in these populations.[10,11,12] The National Society of Genetic Counselors (NSGC) does not currently support use of NIPT in low-risk populations. They suggest that additional clinical validation studies are necessary before NIPT can be used as a first-tier screening modality for all pregnancies.[13]

NIPT became commercially available in October 2012. Shortly after, in December 2012, The American College of Obstetrics and Gynecology published a committee opinion regarding the use of NIPT for fetal aneuploidy.[14] They concluded that NIPT should be offered to patients who have an increased risk for aneuploidy based on age, maternal serum or combined screening results, ultrasound findings, or family history. Further, they stated that cffDNA testing should not be part of routine prenatal laboratory assessment but should be an informed patient choice after pretest counseling. They concluded that NIPT does not replace the accuracy and diagnostic precision of prenatal diagnosis with CVS or amniocentesis, which should remain options for women.

In 2011, a survey of obstetricians revealed that 85% of providers reported a less than high level of knowledge about NIPT.[15] Two years later, a survey of US obstetricians demonstrated an increase in awareness of and knowledge about NIPT, but only 22% of respondents were familiar with NIPT and the associated clinical data.[16] Since the launch of NIPT, we have personally observed that a large percentage of obstetricians referring to our high-risk clinic believe that NIPT is a diagnostic test and counsel their patients as such. It is important to emphasize that although NIPT for aneuploidy is a highly specific and sensitive screen, it is not a diagnostic test. Although this technology analyzes fetal genetic information, it is not considered diagnostic for a variety of reasons. First, the cells are placental in origin and aneuploidy confined to the placenta cannot be distinguished from true fetal aneuploidy with this technology. Second, the presence of extra fetal DNA could be due to a vanishing twin, although technically these cells are expected to clear out of maternal circulation quickly. And third, the results assume that the maternal karyotype is normal; an abnormal maternal karyotype due to cancer or low-level mosaicism significantly affects interpretation of the screening results. The American College of Medical Genetics and Genomics recommends that this testing should be termed Noninvasive Prenatal Screening (NIPS) rather than NIPT, to highlight the limitations of this technology.[17]

NIPT for aneuploidy is likely the beginning of an explosion of prenatal genetic diagnostic possibilities, and with this explosion comes concern for ethical, legal, and practical implications. The

Council for Responsible Genetics published an article regarding the complex issues surrounding the introduction of NIPT(D) into clinical practice.[18] Haymon states that "the ethical and social implications of NIPD are as extensive as its promised applications." Some fear that with the advent of NIPT, prenatal genetic testing will move from the uncommon to the routine. With this comes a need to examine how these tests should be used and what to do with the information gained. Familiar questions of informed consent, abortion, and eugenics have been raised and continue to be topics of heated debate. Some have even suggested that NIPT is a cover-up for modern-day eugenics.[18] Currently practitioners offer genetics-based tests to a select population of women, typically those who have sufficient risk for a fetal condition to warrant offering such testing. Considering the availability of a noninvasive test that may eventually provide patients with a spreadsheet of potential traits and health concerns, eugenics must be considered. With the availability of this information there may be a shift in beliefs of what constitutes a "normal" or desired outcome for a baby. This may change the way that parents view children, shifting from acceptance of what naturally occurs to an idea of customization or design.[19] Patients undergoing genetic counseling reported a strong desire for genetic testing for life-altering medical conditions, but only a minority of patients would consider testing for the purpose of enhancements.[20] However, it is important to recognize that actual behavior often varies once a person is presented with options in a real-life situation. Parents may change what they perceive to be "life-altering" when given the opportunity to test for other conditions. Having not been in a position to choose, it is difficult for parents to know specifically what their choice would be in that hypothetical situation. If such wide-ranging testing became commonplace, parents could be desensitized to the significance of the choices they were being offered.

Greely suggests that the potential for consequences is directly correlated with the accuracy of the test, such that if the test is inaccurate and requires confirmation by amniocentesis its influence will be reduced.[21] Given the high accuracy in the detection of aneuploidy and that the potential exists with this technology for testing of a variety of other conditions/traits with whole genome sequencing, the controversy will be about the uses of NIPT. NIPT is currently available for both sex determination and paternity testing. Prenatal sex determination may be desirable for couples who have an increased risk for having a fetus with a sex-linked or sex-limited condition; however, this technology can also be utilized for nonmedical reasons. For example, couples who prefer one gender over another may choose to have this testing and ultimately may elect to terminate a pregnancy when NIPT reveals the undesired gender. This decision could be motivated by "societal discrimination against females (or males), economic considerations, or family balancing."[22] NIPT for paternity and gender is available as a direct-to-consumer test and therefore does not necessitate clinical guidance.

Prior to the availability of NIPT, prenatal paternity testing was only available via invasive diagnostic testing. Ethicists have argued that NIPT to establish paternity is worrisome, because it may lead to termination of pregnancy if the paternity is uncertain or determined to be that of the undesired candidate. Given the previously discussed limitations of the underlying technology involved in NIPT, this is concerning. Should NIPT technology expand to DNA sequencing, issues of nonpaternity may be inadvertently revealed. Unwanted and unsolicited information such as this has significant and long-lasting implications.[23]

Researchers and commercial laboratories are currently investigating the potential for genetic testing of other fetal conditions, including additional chromosome aberrations and single gene conditions, with use of cffDNA. Although some of the ethical debate is futuristic speculation, there is concern that screening utilizing cffDNA could significantly increase the amount and scope of available prenatal genetic information. This would be especially true if whole fetal genome sequencing becomes available using cffDNA technology. While some information may be helpful for parental reproductive decision making, it is not known how the vast amount of new data may affect such decision making, especially given that the significance of much of what might be learned may not be clearly understood. Although the field of genetics/genomics is ever evolving, the function of greater than 90% of the human coding region is not fully known.[24] Regarding genome sequencing in the prenatal setting, Donley et al state, "Only a small number of the genetic markers that whole genome sequencing will produce have been studied enough to substantiate their connection to disease."[24] In the prenatal setting, identification of variants or alterations, especially when of unknown significance, produces parental fear and anxiety. This can lead to a loss of autonomy and impaired ability to make decisions (BOX 2.1). Additionally, whole-genome analysis may identify genetic susceptibilities for late-onset conditions. If the pregnancy is not terminated, how does this affect the future child's right not to know this information, especially if the information has no medical relevance during childhood? This "anticipatory autonomy right" has been included in the guidelines established for genetic testing in minors in order to protect their autonomy.[25] Since the majority of genetic alterations found in the fetal genome are inherited, fetal genome sequencing may reveal a medical condition or susceptibility to a medical condition in a parent.[26] The true magnitude of ethical considerations cannot be fully appreciated at this time, as the layers of complexity surrounding this technology are just beginning to unfold.

It is clear, however, that each patient who elects to have NIPT should first be provided informed consent. There is published data on what constitutes an informed choice for prenatal testing. Benn et al suggest that informed consent requires that patients are provided with sufficient relevant information and that their decisions are uninfluenced by medical, societal, and political pressures.[27] Any person who is offered NIPT should be counseled regarding the differences between screening and diagnostic testing, the performance of NIPT (sensitivity, specificity, and positive predictive value), a

BOX 2.1 Case Example

Amy was referred to me for genetic counseling at 13 weeks gestation after having a nuchal translucency (NT) ultrasound, which revealed a measurement greater than the 95 percentile, a known risk factor for a fetal chromosome abnormality. During the contracting, Amy reported that her understanding of the appointment was to discuss available testing options for the detection of Down syndrome and also Alzheimer disease. Amy shared that her provider told her about a new blood test which could test for Down syndrome and other genetic conditions.

We began the session by clarifying Amy's statement regarding Alzheimer disease (AD). She reported that her father had early-onset AD and that she would like to have prenatal testing for AD since she was planning to have the new "noninvasive genetic test for Down syndrome anyway." We reviewed the difference between screening and diagnostic testing options. Given her early gestational age, we discussed both chorionic villus sampling (CVS) and amniocentesis, including specific information about the risks, benefits, and limitations of each. We discussed that diagnostic testing is invasive and therefore involves a risk for pregnancy complications, including miscarriage. However, given that these invasive tests obtain intact fetal or placental cells, specific genetic testing can be performed on those cells. With a screening test, a variety of methods are available to provide a pregnancy-specific risk for conditions for which screening is available, but specific conditions cannot be diagnosed or ruled out.

Amy was counseled in detail regarding the ultrasound finding of an increased NT and the possible etiologies, including fetal aneuploidy. We spent time reviewing chromosomes, nondisjunction, and the ultrasound-adjusted risk for fetal aneuploidy. Given this ultrasound finding, Amy was considered to have a "high risk" for fetal aneuploidy. We discussed that CVS (performed at 10–13 weeks gestation) and amniocentesis (performed after 15 weeks gestation) are available for detection of aneuploidy. She understood that chromosome analysis can detect chromosome conditions in which there is an extra or missing chromosome as well as other aberrations (deletions, duplications, inversions, and translocations), but not all genetic conditions. We reviewed that the chromosomes are essentially packages of genes, but that gene alterations are typically too small to be able to be detected cytogenetically. However, if a specific genetic condition is suspected, either by family history or ultrasound findings, individual genes can be analyzed. Given Amy's father's history, we discussed that AD could be tested for with these diagnostic tests. She was counseled that a positive fetal test result would reveal a diagnosis of AD in her. But a negative fetal test result does not change her a priori risk (50%) to have inherited the genetic alteration from her father.

We then reviewed the availability of noninvasive prenatal testing (NIPT). Amy was counseled that this technology analyzes fetal genetic information found in maternal circulation. She understood that while the entire fetal genome can be found in the maternal circulation, most commercial laboratories are currently only analyzing genetic information from select chromosomes (21, 13, 18, X and Y). Thus screening for Down syndrome is available, but analysis for a specific known genetic alteration causing AD is not available by this screening modality. We discussed that in the future this technology will likely become available. We discussed that NIPT detects approximately 99% of cases of Down syndrome in patients

(*continued*)

known to have an increased risk for fetal aneuploidy, with a false-positive rate of approximately 0.1%. She understood that while the sensitivity and specificity are high with this screening option, it is still a screen and the result will be reported as a chance rather than a definitive yes or no. She was also counseled that this technology can identify other information including risks for other aneuploidies and fetal gender.

We also reviewed other screening options including combined screening (first screen), quad screen, and detailed ultrasound. After thoughtful consideration of these options, Amy declined diagnostic testing. She was concerned about the risk for complications and stated that termination of pregnancy is not an option she would consider regardless of genetic test results. She elected to proceed with NIPT and understood that she would be provided with genetic risk information regarding select fetal aneuploidy, not all genetic conditions. She also understood that the NIPT would not provide information regarding the chance for her or her baby to have inherited the familial AD gene change.

priori versus postscreen risks, and the broad spectrum of results and fetal health information that potentially can be obtained (e.g., when screening for Down syndrome, other information regarding risks for trisomy 13, trisomy 18, and sex chromosome aneuploidy may be revealed). These reasons highlight ACOG's recommendation for pretest and posttest genetic counseling. In addition, NSGC released a position statement in January 2013 which also emphasizes the need for genetic counseling. The society urges that "NIPT only be offered in the context of informed consent, education, and counseling by a qualified provider, such as a certified genetic counselor."[13] These recommendations raise another ethical concern, that of access and availability of genetic counseling services. NSGC recognizes that some patients electing to undergo NIPT will not have access to a genetic counselor and recommend that in this scenario, another qualified healthcare professional should provide appropriate pretest counseling to review the current benefits and limitations of the technology.

Prenatal Microarray Analysis

Microarray analysis is a molecular-based technique in which a test sample of DNA is compared to a reference (normal) genome in order to determine if the test sample has any extra or missing DNA. Multiple array platforms exist, each with a variety of benefits and limitations. In recent years this technology has emerged as a frontline diagnostic test for children with congenital anomalies, delayed neurocognitive development, and autism spectrum disorders.[28,29] Microarray analysis has enabled the detection of genomic deletions and duplications that are 100 times smaller than those identified by routine karyotyping. These deletions or duplications, also referred to as *copy number variants* (CNVs), result in genomic variation from the expected DNA content. The effects can be benign, of unknown significance, or clinically significant/pathogenic.[30] Many of these submicroscopic CNVs occur frequently enough to be recognized as specific syndromes (e.g., 22q11 deletion syndrome), while others are previously undescribed.[28] While clinical utility of microarray technology in the postnatal population is widespread, application in the prenatal setting has lagged behind largely because of perceived difficulties in interpreting the results in the context of an ongoing pregnancy.[29]

Stillbirths (fetal death at 20 weeks gestation or greater) occur in approximately 1 in 160 births in the United States[31] and, despite extensive evaluations, the cause of the loss is not discovered in up to 60% of cases.[32] In 2012, Reddy et al investigated the performance of microarray analysis versus standard karyotype analysis in stillborn fetuses. They concluded that microarray analysis is more likely to reveal genomic abnormalities compared with standard karyotyping; the success is in part because microarray analysis can be performed on nonviable tissue but also is due to the detection of pathogenic, submicroscopic CNVs.[33]

The use of microarray analysis in the prenatal setting, however, has been richly debated within the obstetric community. To date, prenatal microarray analysis has been primarily utilized in pregnant women who had a high likelihood of having a fetal chromosome abnormality, including those pregnancies with abnormal ultrasound findings and those with more routine risk factors such as advanced maternal age (AMA) and an abnormal biochemical or combined screening result.[34,35] In 2012, Wapner et al suggested that microarray analysis should be offered as a first tier of prenatal diagnostic testing[31] rather than the more typical karyotype analysis. In determining whether this technology is appropriate as a frontline prenatal test, many factors should be considered including both functional and ethical questions.

Functionally, does microarray analysis identify abnormalities routinely picked up by karyotyping? How commonly are abnormalities discovered by microarray analysis that are missed by standard karyotyping? What percentage of CNVs are significant versus of unknown significance? Wapner et al conducted a large double-blinded prospective study in order to address these questions.[31] The study subjects were women who presented for diagnostic testing via amniocentesis or chorionic villus sampling due to a high risk for fetal aneuploidy (AMA, abnormal serum/combined screening result, abnormal ultrasound findings). Both standard karyotyping and microarray analysis were performed on each sample. Microarray analysis revealed all the aneuploidies and unbalanced genomic aberrations that were identified by karyotype analysis; however, as expected, balanced translocations and triploidy were not detected by microarray analysis. Microarray analysis revealed clinically significant CNVs in approximately 2.5% of fetal samples with normal karyotypes. When these cases were subdivided by indication, about 6% of patients who had an abnormal ultrasound finding and 1.7% of patients who were advanced maternal age (AMA) or had an abnormal screening result had a clinically significant deletion or duplication.[31] This study also demonstrated that about 3.4% of karyotypically normal pregnancies had variants of unknown significance (VUS). Of these, 72.3% had findings that were not easily dismissed as likely to be benign and required expert research to help determine clinical relevance.[31] A variety of earlier prenatal microarray studies found variants of uncertain significance in approximately 0.5%–1.5% of cases studied for a variety of indications.[28,34,36]

With the increased utilization of microarray analysis in both the prenatal and postnatal settings, many databases and genome browsers have been established to help determine the significance of these variants. These include the Database of Chromosomal Imbalance and Phenotype in Humans using Ensembl Resources (DECIPHER), The International Standards for Cytogenomic Arrays (ISCA), Ensembl, and the University of California Santa Cruz (UCSC). These browsers and databases help to determine which genes are included in a specific CNV and, in some cases, genotype-phenotype correlations. As more information is gained and shared with these systems, previously classified VUS will likely be reclassified as either benign or pathogenic.[28,37] In addition, cytogeneticists can aid in the prediction of pathogenicity based on the nature of the variant, whether the variant was inherited or de novo, and by analysis of functional data and/or data about overlapping CNVs reported in other individuals. There are limitations to this approach, and in some cases the significance of the CNVs cannot be elucidated. Other CNVs are not fully penetrant, and the genetic modifiers that predict phenotype are largely unknown at this time. Thus the clinical significance of a variant cannot always be accurately predicted, even when the variant has known potential to be pathogenic.[37] The process of determining the significance of a variant is often time consuming and requires multiple steps. In the prenatal setting, determining clinical relevance must be done in a timely fashion.

There are specific ethical considerations with use of microarray analysis that are unique to the prenatal setting. In this situation, informed consent must not only include a detailed discussion of the purpose of the testing, its coverage of the genome and how that differs from standard karyotyping, but also include examples of the types of changes that can be detected—incidental findings, VUS, nonpaternity, consanguinity—and the conditions with varying degrees of severity that may be detected with this technology.[37] Providing appropriate informed consent should afford patients the opportunity to consider the possible outcomes prior to receiving an unexpected result. In order to allow for such anticipatory guidance and exploration of feelings, both pretest and posttest genetic counseling is recommended.[28,37]

Identification of VUS can cause significant anxiety for both the patient and the provider. Bernhardt et al showed that women who received unclear results had anxiety during and even after delivery, with many regretting having had the testing.[38] While maternal anxiety following prenatal screening has been well documented in the literature,[39] microarray analysis in the prenatal setting opens the door for additional uncertainty and distress. Regarding patient anxiety, McGillvray et al concluded that women should not be denied access to prenatal microarray analysis because of the risk of uncertain results, but rather that patients electing to have such technology should be given adequate pretest and posttest genetic counseling.[37] When delivering results of unknown significance, genetic counselors reported feeling a burden of responsibility.[38] Ethicists have debated that VUS and the resulting maternal/provider anxiety may lead to an unnecessary increase in terminations of pregnancy. However, for those electing to terminate a pregnancy, the severity of the fetal condition is a consistent indicator.[40] Considering this data, variants of unknown significance are unlikely to result in a significant increase in the number of elective terminations.[37] Advances in technology that could potentially result in an increase in elective terminations will remain a topic of controversy between the pro-life and pro-choice groups, and because of this controversy it is necessary that prenatal counseling remain nondirective and respectful of parental values and decisions.[41]

Functional limitations of microarray analysis can be reduced with use of specific array platforms, selected based on the indication for testing and the patient's individual needs. With this technology, the potential exists to test for the presence of variants that may suggest predisposition to adult-onset disorders.

The American College of Obstetrics and Gynecology (ACOG) released a committee opinion in 2009 suggesting that further investigation is necessary in order to determine the usefulness of microarray analysis as a first-line test for prenatal evaluation of chromosome abnormalities.[42] This is primarily due to limitations with detection of balanced chromosome rearrangements and polyploidies, the detection of VUS, and reduced cost effectiveness. They acknowledge that prenatal array can be offered in the setting of an abnormal ultrasound finding and a normal fetal karyotype as well as in cases of fetal demise with congenital anomalies (BOX 2.2), specifically when routine karyotyping is not informative (ACOG committee opinion). The role of microarray analysis in a prenatal setting is evolving and, as such, prenatal microarray analysis is likely to be accepted as first-tier screening not only in anomalous or stillborn fetuses but also in structurally normal fetuses.[28,29]

Expanded Carrier Screening

Ethnic-specific carrier testing has been available for more than 10 years to couples considering a future pregnancy or to couples who are currently pregnant.[43] With the completion of sequencing of the human genome and the availability of next-generation

BOX 2.2 Case Example

Amy was referred to us for genetic counseling at 18 weeks gestation after having a routine detailed anatomy ultrasound, which revealed a congenital heart defect (CHD) and possible cleft palate. Ultrasound was repeated and the fetal findings were confirmed. During the contracting, Amy expressed interest in testing to determine if the fetus has an underlying genetic cause for the anomalies detected by ultrasound.

We counseled Amy regarding each specific anomaly, including the various etiologies. Specifically, we discussed that these findings can be syndromic or nonsyndromic, sporadic or inherited. Additionally, we discussed that these differences can be environmental, multifactorial, or genetic in etiology. Regarding genetic causes, we discussed that the combination of findings could be due to fetal aneuploidy, other chromosome aberrations (deletions, duplications, inversions, and unbalanced chromosome translocations), and single gene conditions. We spent time reviewing chromosomes, nondisjunction, and the ultrasound-adjusted risk for fetal aneuploidy. Given the ultrasound findings, Amy was now considered to have a "high risk" for fetal aneuploidy. We discussed that amniocentesis was available for detection of fetal aneuploidy. She understood that standard chromosome analysis can detect chromosome conditions in which there is an extra or missing chromosome as well as some other large chromosome aberrations, but not all genetic conditions.

We also reviewed the option of prenatal microarray analysis on the fetal cells obtained from amniocentesis. Amy was counseled that prenatal microarray analysis is a test that analyzes the fetal genome by comparing a test sample of DNA (the fetal DNA) to a reference (normal) genome to determine if the test sample has any extra or missing DNA. We reviewed the availability of multiple array platforms. Although this technology is currently standard of care for liveborn children with congenital anomalies as a frontline test (before or in place of standard karyotype), it is often still used as a second-tier test in the prenatal setting following standard chromosome analysis. Amy was counseled that approximately 6% of fetuses with an abnormal ultrasound finding(s) and a normal karyotype have a copy number variant (CNV) detectable by microarray analysis. She was counseled at length regarding the benefits and limitations of microarray analysis as well as the broad range of possible results that could be obtained from such technology, including changes suggestive of adult-onset disorders, variants of unknown significance, nonpaternity, and consanguinity.

After thoughtful consideration of these options and extensive pretest counseling, Amy elected to have amniocentesis with standard chromosome analysis. She elected to follow up with prenatal microarray analysis if the karyotype was within normal limits. A specific targeted microarray platform was selected to minimize undesired results.

sequencing methods, the carrier screening paradigm is beginning to shift from ancestry-based to a process that screens for many disorders at one time.[44] Several commercial laboratories are currently offering screening for multiple disorders using a single blood sample. This is referred to as *expanded carrier screening* (ECS). Given that the cost of ECS rivals that of single-gene carrier screening, ECS is gaining attention among reproductive healthcare providers. Although there are perceived benefits to ECS, primarily those of decreasing the incidence of inherited genetic disease, many concerns exist regarding widespread integration of ECS into routine prenatal care.[43] The current lack of professional guidelines about the use of ECS lends uncertainty regarding to whom this technology should be offered. Surveyed genetics professionals expressed concerns about the specific mutations for the conditions evaluated by ECS and the applicability of the tested gene alterations to all ethnic groups. Further, this group worried that reproductive healthcare providers may not follow up with an abnormal ECS result in the most appropriate manner (e.g., offering the best follow-up testing option to the partner).[43]

To date, there is limited input from professional organizations regarding the specific genes and mutations to include in ECS panels. As such, the American College of Medical Genetics and Genomics (ACMG) released a policy statement in March 2013 to address concerns regarding ECS. They suggest that "selection of appropriate disease-causing targets for general population-based carrier screening should be developed using clear criteria, rather than simply including as many disorders as possible."[44]

The ACMG published specific criteria that should be met when laboratories are considering which disorders to include in expanded carrier screening panels. These state:

1. Disorders should be of a nature that carriers would consider having prenatal testing.
2. When adult-onset disorders are included, patients considering testing must provide informed consent, since identification of such a gene alteration may have implications to the person undergoing screening or her/his family members.
3. For each disorder, the causative gene(s), mutations, and carrier frequencies should be known, so that residual risk can be assessed.
4. There must be validated clinical association between the mutations(s) tested for and the severity of the disorder.

5. There must be compliance with the American College of Medical Genetics and Genomics Standards and Guidelines for Clinical Genetics Laboratories, including quality control and proficiency testing.[44]

Obtaining informed consent for ECS presents challenges to the provider since each disease in the multidisease screening panel cannot be discussed with the same detail as that typically provided with single-condition screening. Patients considering ECS should be provided with written information on the conditions for which the screening panel tests and should be given the opportunity to review this information prior to proceeding with the testing. Both pretest and posttest counseling should be made available to the patient electing to have ECS. Research has shown that reproductive healthcare providers receive limited training in the field of genetics[45,46]; therefore, providers offering ECS should work closely with genetic counselors or medical geneticists.[43]

Genetic counselors are accustomed to discussing the conditions for which a couple may have an increased risk because of their ancestry. It can be overwhelming when there are other, potentially more pressing issues to address. It is considered standard of care to offer sickle cell anemia screening to African-American families and screening for cystic fibrosis to Caucasian families. But to have to discuss 100 conditions or more, including the carrier frequency (which may or may not be known) and the detection rate, is an impossible task. Not only is there not enough time allocated, one cannot expect patients to adequately absorb that information in a way that allows for truly *informed* consent. Thus, counselors are left to do the best they can with little or no guidance as to what constitutes adequate counseling. Preconception may be a better time to broach this subject with a genetic counselor. At that time, there is not the same urgency that may exist in pregnancy.

Clearly there are ethical issues scattered throughout the realm of prenatal counseling and screening. When considering the application of ethical principles to prenatal genetics and prenatal genetic counseling, we have to consider to whom these principles should be directed. Is our focus the pregnant patient? Should we be considering the fetus as our patient? Or the couple as a unit? The way in which one should ethically act may depend upon the perspective from which we are looking. Certainly, as in medicine, the genetic counselor's role is to do good for his or her patient, do no harm, and respect his or her autonomy while providing nondirective counseling. These principles are inexorably linked.

Autonomy is defined as the right or capacity to make one's own rational decisions. Unless shown or known to be otherwise, pregnant women can be assumed to have the decision-making capacity to make their own assessments related to their medical care and that of their unborn babies. There will always be situations in which an individual has limited capacity for understanding, which would of course be an exception and require different management. Like all persons, a pregnant woman's decisions are made based on her own value system, life experiences, and beliefs. The value system of the genetic counselor is irrelevant. The principle of autonomy tells us that a prenatal patient considering testing, screening, termination, or continuation of a pregnancy must be able to act on her own decisions without coercion or influence from her genetic counselor or other care provider. In order for a patient to exercise her autonomy, though, she must first be provided complete and unbiased information about all available choices (informed consent). A genetic counselor can unintentionally limit a patient's autonomy by not offering a particular test to her if, for example, the genetic counselor feels that the information will overwhelm the patient such that she becomes confused. If a patient presents in the first trimester for genetic counseling, depending upon her risk factors she could be offered screening by way of first screen, cell-free fetal DNA, quad screen, first trimester ultrasound, and/or second trimester ultrasound. She could also be offered carrier screening based on her ethnicity (cystic fibrosis, sickle cell anemia, spinal muscular atrophy, alpha thalassemia, beta thalassemia, fragile X syndrome, Tay Sachs disease, etc.) or an expanded carrier screen. She could be offered diagnostic testing by way of amniocentesis or CVS, including a discussion of chromosome analysis, AFAFP analysis, and even microarray testing. And this is what would be offered without any exceptional concerns or risk factors. How can one patient be expected to understand and be able to make an autonomous decision when presented with this many options? This information is challenging for those with a college degree; what about those with just a high school diploma or less, or those for whom English is not their first language?

A genetic counselor may not make a particular test available to a patient because it is not in the typical realm of tests offered. Thinking about our case scenario (BOX 2.3), how would this have been different if Amy was 36 years old, came for genetic counseling because of age, and simply shared this family history? If a provider were not to offer her prenatal testing for the adult-onset Alzheimer disease, would he or she be preventing her from exercising her autonomy by not offering all available options? Prenatal testing is technically available for known DNA mutations but is not typically provided prenatally for adult-onset conditions. In fact, the American College of Medical Genetics (ACMG) and National Society of Genetic Counselors (NSGC) Joint Practice Guidelines on Genetic Counseling and Testing for Alzheimer Disease states that "Prenatal testing for Alzheimer disease is not advised if the patient intends to continue a pregnancy with a mutation."[47] Genetic counselors are bound to act by the code of ethics and practice guidelines of their governing organizations (NSGC and ABGC, the American Board of Genetic Counseling). When there are position statements indicating that certain testing is not appropriate or not to be offered (such as presymptomatic testing of pediatric patients for adult-onset disorders), then a genetic counselor should not counsel a family about such testing. Following this pattern of thought, if Amy would consider

BOX 2.3 Case Example

Amy was referred for genetic counseling at 16 weeks gestation for amniocentesis, but the referral information sent did not identify what the indication for amniocentesis was. During the contracting phase of the conversation, we inquired what her indication was for amniocentesis. She reported that her primary obstetrician had told her to come for genetic counseling and amniocentesis after she expressed concern over her father's diagnosis of early-onset Alzheimer disease. Amy reported that she wanted to have amniocentesis in order to know if her baby would be likely to develop early-onset Alzheimer disease.

We reviewed prenatal testing by way of amniocentesis including the risks, benefits, and limitations of this testing option. We discussed that while the likelihood of not having any complication following the procedure is significantly greater than the chance for a complication or fetal loss, there is still a real risk and care needs to be taken in determining if this risk is acceptable to her.

We spent the next several minutes reviewing Amy's family history and that of her husband. This revealed that Amy's father has Alzheimer disease (AD), had genetic testing performed, and a mutation was identified. To date, however, Amy has not had testing for this mutation, which she has a 50% chance to carry. We discussed that if she were to have the same gene mutation as her father, this does not guarantee that she will develop AD. Similarly, if her child were to have the mutation, the susceptibility allele may never have a clinical consequence for her child. As she has not had testing, there is a 25% (1 in 4) chance (1/2 chance for her to have inherited it and 1/2 chance for her to pass it on) for each of her children to inherit the gene mutation her father has. Conversely, there is a 75% chance (3 in 4) for each child not to inherit the gene mutation.

We decided that it would be useful to examine Amy's motivation and intention in seeking prenatal testing and to try to elucidate if it was her idea or that of her care provider or another family member. We discussed that when considering prenatal testing or prenatal screening, one must take into account what the goal of the screening or testing is. That is, does Amy want to know what her risk is so that she can act upon it during pregnancy? We discussed that for some people, acting upon results would mean termination of pregnancy, but for others it can mean alternative management of pregnancy based upon new information. We discussed an example: if a fetus is diagnosed with Down syndrome prenatally, there is a recommendation for fetal echocardiogram because 50% of babies with Down syndrome have heart defects. In addition, some parents may want to learn all they can about Down syndrome and meet other families who have a child with Down syndrome, or deliver at a larger community hospital. Other families may elect to terminate the pregnancy upon learning of the diagnosis. We discussed this hypothetical scenario with Amy to help her start to ask herself these questions (if she had not already done so). It was important for Amy to ask herself: if she learned that her fetus had inherited the AD mutation from her and her father, what would that mean for her pregnancy? As AD is an adult-onset condition, this presymptomatic diagnosis would not alter the management for Amy or her fetus during pregnancy. It would also not be information relevant to this child during its youth. Additionally, because a positive test result in her fetus would mean she also had the gene mutation, how would learning her

(*continued*)

own diagnosis during her pregnancy impact her? Would this be the most appropriate way to find out about her increased risk for developing AD? Finally, we discussed whether knowing at 16 weeks of pregnancy would be relevant to her. Does she need to know now so that she can more safely terminate the pregnancy at an earlier gestation, or would finding out this information later in pregnancy, or even after delivery, be just as beneficial? We discussed each of these hypothetical situations, allowing for consideration of the benefits and risks of each option. Is her need to know at 16 weeks greater than her concern over the risk of fetal loss at 16 weeks?

There are many factors that go into the decision-making process. It is the genetic counselor's responsibility to enable Amy to exercise her autonomy in a meaningful way in the informed consent process. We need to provide complete information in a way that does not bias or overwhelm Amy. We decided it was important to spend some time discussing the NSGC (National Society of Genetic Counselors) and ACMG (American College of Medical Genetics and Genomics) joint practice guidelines for testing for AD.[47] These organizations laid out a model for predictive testing which begins with neurological, neuropsychological, and psychiatric evaluation prior to the initiation of testing. If she were to have prenatal testing for AD, she would be skipping these crucial steps. For this reason, Amy elected not to proceed with amniocentesis at the time of our initial meeting. She did not have another indication for this testing and knew that she was not in a place to have predictive testing herself or to learn about her own status. Amy stated that she had not considered what a positive result would mean in terms of her own status and was not ready to come to terms with that result right now.

termination of pregnancy, do the guidelines suggest that testing for AD should be offered to her? And should she have to make that decision prior to a discussion about prenatal testing?

Decisions about termination of pregnancy need to be made without any coercive influence from others. This extends to the genetic counselor, other healthcare providers, and family members. A genetic counselor's personal feelings may be easy to mask when the conversation is about cell-free fetal DNA, but can be more difficult to hide when the discussion surrounds the termination of a previable or viable fetus. It is actually the genetic counselor's role and responsibility to advocate on behalf of the woman's expressed wishes and ensure her autonomy. That brings up the issue of the autonomy of the fetus. What if the parents wanted to have testing for an adult-onset condition? Doesn't this future child (future adult) have the right not to know? The purpose of prenatal testing is not necessarily to "offer limitless insight into the genetic make-up of a future child."[48]

Informed consent is the process by which a patient is fully informed such that she can exercise her autonomy in choices about her health care. When a woman is pregnant, that extends to making decisions about her pregnancy and unborn baby. It is widely accepted that there are several components to the informed consent process. First, the patient must recognize that there is a decision to be made and that whichever choice she makes is good and reasonable. Second, the genetic counselor must provide details about each available option including the risks, benefits, and limitations of each, together with the possible outcomes of each. For example, a patient could elect either to have noninvasive prenatal testing (NIPT) or amniocentesis. In addition to discussing the risks, benefits, and limitations of each test, it would be important to discuss that she could have a normal result, an abnormal result, or no result. She could also have a result regarding a condition about which she was not previously concerned (for example, she had testing because she was concerned about an increased risk for trisomy 18, a severe condition, and learns the baby has triple X syndrome). The third step is recognizing if the patient understands this information. This can be ensured not only by asking if the information is clear and what questions the patient has, but also by asking the patient to retell what has been told to her. She could be asked how she would explain this to her partner, mother, or friend who is not present. This allows the genetic counselor to assess the patient's level of understanding and to clarify any confusing information or misunderstandings.

An example of such confusion occurred with a patient who was carrying a baby who had been diagnosed with an encephalocele. Ultrasound demonstrated that half of the contents of the brain were in a sac protruding from the skull. The providers knew that this meant that the fetus had less than adequate brain tissue, as the brain tissue in the encephalocele was disorganized and dysplastic and therefore nonfunctional. The patient indicated that she understood what she was told about the lack of normal brain tissue present. However, upon repeating the information, she indicated that she was reassured because none of the normal brain tissue was present in the encephalocele. That way if surgery was performed postnatally, the baby would not be losing any normal brain tissue. She heard that the brain tissue in the encephalocele was all abnormal; thus, after surgery, only abnormal tissue would be absent. All of the normal tissue would remain intact inside the cranium. She interpreted this as though the tissue inside the encephalocele was not normal and therefore extra and not necessary. In her mind, then, removing the encephalocele would not remove necessary, normal brain tissue and would leave her baby with only normal brain tissue, which was all it needed. She heard the information as it was expressed, but based on her own history, education, and life experiences, the same words had different meaning for her. In this situation, allowing her to retell the information revealed the confusion and presented an opportunity to clarify. The fourth component of informed consent is when the patient makes a voluntary decision. Thus, the ultimate decision the patient makes is also part of the informed consent process that she is able to come to an autonomous decision. A decision to consent to or decline a screening or diagnostic test, based upon her values, beliefs, and life experiences, is the ultimate goal of the process.

Prenatal genetic counseling is designed to enable a woman to exercise her autonomy in the informed consent process. Sometimes in this process, a woman is simply unable to make a decision. It may be that she needs to seek counsel from a trusted advisor, spouse, religious or spiritual mentor, family member, or friend. This conversation can be done privately, after the visit, or the patient may prefer to include the genetic counselor to allow for further interpretation and explanation. Alternatively, the patient may instead decide to return at a later time to review further the options available to her. However, it is important for her to be aware that *not* making a decision is also a choice. As declining all available testing options is one choice available to her, not making a decision as to how to proceed is, in effect, deciding to not pursue testing, at least for that moment. Some patients may respond to the prenatal testing options by declining even to hear about the assessment of risk. Others may elect to pursue some form of testing. As discussed, still others may be uncertain about what to do next. Just as important as counseling regarding the risks and benefits is counseling about the timing of such tests. Delaying a decision may mean that a woman can no longer have a particular test. A component of counseling is informing the patient that there is a window of time that first trimester screening, CVS, and quad screen are available. Other tests do not have such gestational age–related restrictions. However, there may be limitations as to what can be done with the results of such testing. Termination of pregnancy is currently a legal option in every state, but the gestational age at which the procedure can be legally performed and the legal indications vary by state. It is an important component of the prenatal genetic counseling process to discuss termination, including the legal limits as defined by state law and other states whose laws may be different.

During the genetic counseling process, a woman may indicate that termination is not an option for her regardless of the fetal diagnosis. However, any genetic counselor who has provided prenatal counseling will have numerous examples of patients who have been certain of what they would do given a particular scenario and who have later changed their minds completely when they have come face to face with that diagnosis and option. In more than one situation a prenatal genetic counselor will encounter a couple who is adamantly opposed to termination of pregnancy and will state that outright. However, a short time later, when they are faced with a devastating or lethal diagnosis, they may change their minds. Conversely, couples may state that they are certain they would elect to end a pregnancy if an anomaly was found. However, upon hearing the diagnosis and learning about it, or realizing they are attached more strongly to the fetus than they thought they would be, they choose to continue the pregnancy. An interesting example was when a couple was seen for genetic counseling for an increased Down syndrome risk through maternal serum screening. After receiving genetic counseling, the woman consented to amniocentesis because the parents felt that they needed to know if their baby had Down syndrome, so they could make a decision about continuing or ending the pregnancy. The results of the amniocentesis revealed Down syndrome. At the initial genetic counseling visit, the couple had stated that they would terminate the pregnancy if they learned that the baby had Down syndrome. They felt that it would be more than they could manage to raise a child with that condition. Following the diagnosis, they were scheduled for a fetal echocardiogram to evaluate further the health-related issues in their baby. After learning that the baby's heart appeared normal, the wife turned to her husband and said, "So can we keep him?" Her husband said, "Oh yes, of course we can." During the testing process they had both reconsidered their opinions about Down syndrome and about termination, but had never said anything to each other about it. These are not families that are coerced into changing their minds; they are families who realize that sometimes reality is different than what they expected it would be. Most individuals believe that they know what they would do when faced with a particular set of circumstances. However, if they have never had to make that decision before, with the current set of circumstances, they may respond differently. For this reason, it is essential in not only ensuring patient autonomy, but also in providing complete informed consent to discuss all options and potential outcomes. Informed consent, in essence, requires information presented at a level that the patient can understand in an environment that supports good decision making. It also requires active support of and respect for the patient's right to make that decision. Informed consent promotes and protects patient autonomy and is an ongoing and evolving process, not one with a fixed ending.

Beneficence and nonmaleficence are related concepts in the realm of ethics and medicine. **Beneficence** suggests that one should act in such a way that beneficial results are produced. Usually in health care, beneficence is interpreted as a healthcare professional's duty to act in a manner that in his or her best judgment will benefit the patient. It also refers to an action that is done for the benefit of others. **Nonmaleficence** means to do no harm. Healthcare providers are expected to refrain from causing harm, but also to provide care that helps their patients. Striking a balance between these two can be challenging in prenatal genetics. Invasive testing can potentially lead to fetal loss, which would certainly cause harm to the fetus as a patient but also emotional and physical harm to the parent(s). However, some may see the birth of a child with anomalies as a burden to that child or to his or her parents or family unit. Thus, the burden of this child's medical issues could cause harm such that the termination of this pregnancy could be considered a beneficent act. By extension, offering of prenatal testing and screening would be beneficent. However, all screening tests carry with them a risk for increased anxiety, with either a false-positive or false-negative result. As there are degrees of harm as well as perception of harm, the principle of a patient's autonomy helps to define which would be "more harmful" to her. Many prenatal genetic counselors try to assess this by asking a patient considering amniocentesis because of the risk for a fetal chromosome condition "which, of two unlikely outcomes, would be more difficult for you: the birth of child with this condition and you didn't know it, or the loss of a healthy pregnancy due to a procedure-related complication?" Historically, these ethical principles were based on the traditional doctor–patient relationship that was customarily paternalistic. Genetic counseling is quite different from that traditional use of medicine. A genetic counselor's respect for maternal autonomy supersedes these other ethical principles in many respects.

Nonmaleficence extends to making sure that no harm is done in the beneficent act of using new technology that has not been well studied. For example: a patient comes for prenatal testing by amniocentesis because her father has an X-linked recessive condition with a known detectable mutation. After counseling regarding the genetics of X-linked conditions and her status as an obligate carrier and after completing the informed consent process, she undergoes amniocentesis. The ultrasound indicates that this is a male fetus and, as such, would have a 50% chance of having received the deleterious mutation. As a matter of routine, to rule out maternal cell contamination, a maternal blood sample is sent to the reference lab with the amniotic fluid. The results on the fetus are returned and indicate that the male fetus does not have the known mutation in the family. There is a notation at the bottom of the report indicating that the laboratory also tested the maternal blood sample and she does not have the familial mutation. She is an obligate carrier because her father has this X-linked condition, and she would have had to have received his X chromosome to be female, but she does not have the mutation—thus, nonpaternity has been revealed. She has not requested nor consented for paternity testing for herself, but now the information exists. She has the right not to know (as she didn't ask the question). Would the medical professionals in the case be doing more harm by not telling her and potentially subjecting her to further amniocentesis in future pregnancies for a risk that does not exist? The principle of beneficence refers to the moral obligation to act for the benefit of others. One could say that beneficence in genetic counseling refers to the genetic counselor's perspective on the health-related interests of the patient. In prenatal genetic counseling, who is your patient? Is it the woman or her fetus? Is it the couple or all of them as a family? When we introduce these concepts back into Amy's family, we see that if one is to identify what characterizes the promotion of health over harm we need to know whose health and whose harm is being considered.

The prenatal realm of genetics is rich with ethical dilemmas. If one just looks at Amy's small family history, the areas for ethical debate are plentiful. There is the issue of prenatal testing for an adult-onset disease, presymptomatic testing, and termination of pregnancy for an adult-onset disorder. When we look to the obvious ethical principles for guidance, the path is still not clear. Pregnancy is an overwhelming and stressful time in general. We can infer that Amy is concerned about her father and overwhelmed by his care. In addition, she has a young child and is pregnant. She is concerned about the inevitable loss of her father and knowing the toll his illness is taking on herself and her family. She may worry about what that will do to her children. She likely wants to avoid placing a burden on them with (the risk for) her own illness, but may also want to avoid the guilt of passing on this condition to them. Michael may have a completely different agenda; but are his wishes even considered when Amy is the one who is pregnant, and ultimately she is able to make decisions for her own body?

Many care providers or patients view prenatal testing and screening as something, in part at least, for which there must be justification. "I need to know because I won't continue the pregnancy," or "I need to know so I won't worry during the rest of the pregnancy," or "I need to know so that I can be prepared and deliver at a different hospital." Others believe that making a diagnosis prenatally is an ethical responsibility in order to ensure that a child is healthy. In this case they may believe that to decline testing requires an explanation: "it wouldn't matter to us either way," or "it is not worth the risk of the procedure," or "it can't be fixed and it will just make me worry." Autonomy, informed consent, nondirectiveness, nonmaleficence, and beneficence are important practices to uphold. However, some of the time that is easier said than done. In many instances in prenatal genetic counseling, these tenets are in opposition to each other. At times, the question may be in regard to when the fetus has its own moral position. Do the rights of the parents overrule the rights of the fetus? Genetic counselors providing prenatal counseling have to, at the same time, ensure reproductive autonomy for the woman and her partner, provide parental informed consent for testing as well as declination of testing, and consider the beneficence toward the fetus as a (potential) future child.

REFERENCES

1. Bianchi, D.W., Mahr, A., Zickwolf, G.K., Houseal, T.W., Flint, A.F., Klinger, K.W. (1992). Detection of fetal cells with 47,XY,+21 karyotype in maternal peripheral blood. *Human Genetics*. 90(4):368–370.
2. Lo, Y.M., Corbetta, N., Chamberlain, P.F., Rai, V., Sargent, I.L., Redman, C.W. (1997). Presence of fetal DNA in maternal plasma and serum. *Lancet*. 350(9076):485–487.
3. Norton, M.E., Brar, H., Weiss, J., Karimi, A., Laurent, L.C., Caughey, A.B., et al. (2012). Non-Invasive Chromosomal Evaluation (NICE) Study: Results of a multicenter prospective cohort study for detection of fetal trisomy 21 and trisomy 18. *American Journal of Obstetrics & Gynecology*. 207(2):e1–e8.
4. Ashoor, G., Syngelaki, A., Wagner, M., Birdir, C., Nicolaides, K.H. (2012). Chromosome-selective sequencing of maternal plasma cell-free DNA for first-trimester detection of trisomy 21 and trisomy 18. *American Journal of Obstetrics & Gynecology*. 206(322) e.1–e5.
5. Palomaki, G.E., Kloza, E.M., Lambert-Messerlian, G.M., Haddow, J.E., Neveux, L.M., Ehrich, M., et al. (2011). DNA sequencing of maternal plasma to detect Down syndrome: an

international clinical validation study. *Genetics in Medicine.* 13(11):913–920.

6. Bianchi, D.W., Platt, L.D., Goldberg, J.D., Abuhamad, A.Z., Sehnert, A.J., Rava, R.P. (2012). Genome-Wide fetal aneuploidy detection by maternal plasma DNA sequencing. *Obstetrics & Gynecology.* 119(5):890–901.
7. Zimmerman, B., Hill, M., Gemelos, G., Demko, Z., Banjevic, M., Baner, J., et al. (2012). Noninvasive prenatal aneuploidy testing of chromosomes 13, 18, 21, X and Y, using targeted sequencing of polymorphic loci. *Prenatal Diagnosis.* 32(13):1233–1241.
8. Mazloom, A.R., Dzakula, Z., Oeth, P., Wang, H., Jensen, T., Tynan, J., et al. (2013). Noninvasive prenatal detection of sex chromosomal aneuploidies by sequencing circulating cell-free DNA from maternal plasma. *Prenatal Diagnosis.* 33(6):591–597.
9. Nicolaides, K.H., Syngelaki, A., Gil, M., Atanasova, V., Markova, D. (2013). Validation of targeted sequencing of single-nucleotide polymorphisms for non-invasive prenatal detection of aneuploidy of chromosomes 13, 18, 21, X, and Y. *Prenatal Diagnosis.* 33(6):575–579.
10. Canick, J.A., Kloza, E.M., Lambert-Messerlian, G.M., Haddow, J.E., Ehrich, M., van den Boom, D., et al. (2012). DNA Sequencing of maternal plasma to identify Down syndrome and other trisomies in multiple gestations. *Prenatal Diagnosis* 32(8):730–734.
11. Srinivasan, A., Bianchi, D., Liao, W., Sehnert, A., Rava, R. (2013). Maternal plasma DNA sequencing: effects of multiple gestation on aneuploidy detection and the relative cell-free fetal DNA (cffDNA) per fetus. *American Journal of Obstetrics & Gynecology.* 208:S31.
12. Nicolaides, K.H., Syngelaki, A., Ashoor, G., Birdir, C., Touzet, G. (2012). Noninvasive prenatal testing for fetal trisomies in a routinely screened first-trimester population. *American Journal of Obstetrics & Gynecology.* 207(374):e1–e6.
13. National Society of Genetic Counselors. www.nsgc.org
14. American College of Obstetricians and Gynecologists Committee on Genetics. (2012). Committee Opinion No. 545: Noninvasive prenatal testing for fetal aneuploidy. *Obstetrics and Gynecology.* 120(6):1532–1534.
15. Sayres, L.C., Allyse, M., Norton, M.E., Cho, M.K. (2011). Cell-free fetal DNA testing: a pilot study of obstetric healthcare provider

attitudes toward clinical implementation. *Prenatal Diagnosis.* 31(11):1070–1076.

16. Musci, T.J., Fairbrother, G., Batey, A., Bruursema, J., Struble, C., Song, K. (2013). Non-invasive prenatal testing with cell-free DNA: US physician attitudes toward implementation in clinical practice. *Prenatal Diagnosis.* 33(5):424–428.
17. Gregg, A.R., Gross, S.J., Best, R.G., Monaghan, K.G., Bajaj, K., Skotko, B.G., et al. (2013). ACMG statement on noninvasive prenatal screening for fetal aneuploidy. *Genetics in Medicine.* 15(5):395–398.
18. Haymon, L. (2011). Genewatch: The Fast and the Furious. Retrieved from http://www.councilforresponsiblegenetics.org/GeneWatch/GeneWatchPage.aspx?pageId=352.
19. Sandel, M.J. (2007). *The Case against Perfection: Ethics in the Age of Genetic Engineering.* Cambridge: Harvard University Press.
20. Hathaway, F., Burns, E., Ostrer, H. (2009). Consumers' desire towards current and prospective reproductive genetic testing. *Journal of Genetic Counseling.* 18(2):137–146.
21. Greely, H.T. (2011). Get ready for the flood of fetal gene screening. *Nature.* 469(7330):289–291.
22. Benn, P.A., Chapman, A.R. (2010). Ethical challenges in providing noninvasive prenatal diagnosis. *Current Opinion in Obstetrics and Gynecology.* 22(2):128–134.
23. Newsome, A.J. (2008). Ethical aspects arising from noninvasive fetal diagnosis. *Seminars in Fetal & Neonatal Medicine.* 13(2):103–108.
24. Donley, G., Hull, S.C., Berkman, B.E. (2012). Prenatal whole genome sequencing: just because we can, should we? *The Hasting Center Report.* 42(4):28–40.
25. Feinberg, J. (1980). The Child's Right to an Open Future. In: Aiken, W., LaFollete, H., eds. *Whose Child? Children's Rights, Parental Authority, and State Power* (pp. 124–153). Totowa, New Jersey: Rowman and Littlefield.
26. Netzer, C., Schmitz, D., Henn, W. (2012). To know or not to know the genetic sequence of a fetus. *Nature Reviews. Genetics.* 13(10):3333.
27. Benn, P., Cuckle, H., Pergament, E. (2013). Non-invasive prenatal testing for aneuploidy: current status and future prospects. *Ultrasound in Obstetrics & Gynecology.* 42(1):15–33.

28. Savage, M.S., Mourad, M.J., Wapner, R.J. (2011). Evolving applications of microarray analysis in prenatal diagnosis. *Current Opinion in Obstetrics and Gynecology.* 23(2):103–108.
29. Callaway, J.L., Shaffer, L.G., Chitty, L.S., Rosenfeld, J.A., Crolla, J.A. (2013). The clinical utility of microarray technologies applied to prenatal cytogenetics in the presence of a normal conventional karyotype: a review of the literature. *Prenatal Diagnosis.* 33(12):1119–1123.
30. Wapner, R.J., Martin, C.L., Levy, B., Ballif, B.C., Eng, C.M., Zachary, J.M., et al. (2012). Chromosomal Microarray versus karyotyping for prenatal diagnosis. *New England Journal of Medicine.* 367(23):2175–2184.
31. MacDorman, M.F. and Kirmeyer, S. (2009). Fetal and perinatal mortality, United States 2005. *National Vital Statistics Report.* 57(8):1–19.
32. Smith, G.C., Fretts, R.C. (2007). Stillbirth. *Lancet.* 370(9600): 1715–1725.
33. Reddy, U.M., Page, G.P., Saade, G.R., Silver, R.M., Thorsten, V.R., Parker, C.B., et al. (2012). Karyotype versus microarray testing for genetic abnormalities. *New England Journal of Medicine.* 367(23):2185–2193.
34. Coppinger, J., Alliman, S., Lamb, A.N., Torchia, B.S., Bejjani, B.A., Shaffer, L.G. (2009). Whole-genome microarray analysis in prenatal specimens identifies clinically significant chromosome alterations without increase in results of unclear significance compared to targeted microarray. *Prenatal Diagnosis.* 29(12):1156–1166.
35. Maya, I., Davidov, B., Gershovitz, L., Zalzstein, Y., Taub, E., Coppinger, J., et al. (2010). Diagnostic utility of array-based comparative genomic hybridization (aCGH) in a prenatal setting. *Prenatal Diagnosis.* 30(12–13):1131–1137.
36. McGillivray, G., Rosenfeld, J.A., McKinlay Gardner, R.J., Gillam, L.H. (2012). Genetic counseling and ethical issues with chromosome microarray analysis in prenatal testing. *Prenatal Diagnosis.* 32(4):389–395.
37. Bernhardt, B., Soucier, D., Hanson, K., et al. (2011). It's a little bit of a black box: patient and provider experiences with the uncertainties of prenatal microarray testing [abstract]. In: *ACMG Annual Clinical Genetics Meeting.* Vancouver, Canada.

38. Baillie, C., Smith, J., Hewison, J., Mason, G. (2000). Ultrasound screening for chromosomal abnormality: Women's reactions to false positive results. *British Journal of Health Psychology.* 5(4):377–394.
39. Marteau, T.M. (1995). Towards informed decisions about prenatal testing: a review. *Prenatal Diagnosis.* 15(13):1215–1226.
40. Shuster, E. (2007). Microarray genetic screening: a prenatal roadblock for life? *Lancet* 369(9560):526–529.
41. ACOG American College of Obstetricians and Gynecologist Committee. (2009). Committee Opinion No. 446: Array comparative genomic hybridization in prenatal diagnosis. *Obstetrics & Gynecology.* 114(5):1161–1163.
42. Cho, D., McGowan, M.L., Metcalfe, J., Sharp, R.R. (2013). Expanded carrier screening in reproductive healthcare: perspectives from genetics professionals. *Human Reproduction.* 28(6):1725–1730.
43. Resta, R. (2013). Screening everyone for everything: a changing model of screening for carrier status of genetic disease. Retrieved from: http://thednaexchange.com/2013/02/20/screening-everyone-for-everything-a-changing-model-of-screening-for-carrier-status-of-genetic-diseases.
44. Grody, W.W., Thompson, B.H, Gregg, A.R., Bean, L.H., Monaghan, K.G., Schneider A., Lebo, R.V. (2013). ACMG position statement on prenatal/preconception expanded carrier screening. *Genetics in Medicine.* 15(6):482–483.
45. Firth, H.V., Lindenbaum, R.H. (1992). UK clinicians' knowledge of and attitudes to the prenatal diagnosis of single gene disorders. *Journal of Medical Genetics.* 29(1):20–23.
46. Macri, C.J., Gaba, N.D., Sitzer, L.M., Freese, L., Bathgate, S.L., Larsen, Jr. J.W. (2005). Implementation and evaluation of a genetics curriculum to improve obstetrician-gynecologist residents' knowledge and skills in genetic diagnosis and counseling. *American Journal of Obstetrics & Gynecology.* 193(5):1794–1797.
47. Goldman, J.S., Hahn, S.E., Catania, J.W., LaRusse-Eckert, S., Butson, M.B., Rumbaugh, M., et al. (2011). Genetic counseling and testing for Alzheimer disease: joint practice guidelines of the American College of Medical Genetics and the National Society of Genetic Counselors. *Genetics in Medicine.* 13(6):597–605.
48. Bunnik, E.M., De Jong, A., Nijsingh, N., De Wert, G.M.W.R. (2013). The new genetics and informed consent: differentiating choice to preserve autonomy. *Bioethics.* 27(6):348–355.

3

The "ART" of Assisted Reproductive Technologies

SONJA EUBANKS HIGGINS

Introduction

Because genetic counselors help to diagnosis and identify genetic conditions in families, they are often in the position of answering a family's questions about ways to prevent genetic conditions in future generations. Options include choosing not to have children, adopting in order to avoid a genetic condition, or choosing to have prenatal diagnosis to determine if a fetus is affected with a condition in the family and then making the difficult decision about whether to continue the pregnancy if the fetus is affected. However, people are increasingly turning to assisted reproductive technologies (ARTs) and preimplantation genetic diagnosis (PGD) to have children free of genetic conditions that occur in the family. The identification of causative genes for many genetic conditions in recent years, as well as the advances in ARTs, has allowed more people to benefit from these technologies. Many people prefer this approach because it allows a couple to start a pregnancy knowing the child will not be affected with the condition in the family, rather than waiting for prenatal diagnosis and then making decisions about whether to continue a pregnancy. However, as with other technologies, an increase in use has led to a new set of ethical questions. This chapter will describe the ethical issues that have developed with clinical use of these technologies.

Background

The Centers for Disease Control and Prevention (CDC), based on the Fertility Clinic Success Rate and Certification Act passed by the US Congress in 1992, defines ARTs as any fertility treatments that involve the manipulation of *both* egg and sperm cells to result in a pregnancy.[1] Based on this definition some fertility treatments—such as intrauterine insemination (IUI), which only involves the manipulation of sperm by inserting them directly into the uterus with a catheter—do not fit the definition. Procedures that do fit the definition include in vitro fertilization (IVF), gamete intrafallopian transfer (GIFT), zygote intrafallopian transfer (ZIFT) and frozen embryo transfer (FET).[1,2] By far the most commonly used of these treatments is IVF, typically used by couples experiencing infertility as well as those desiring PGD. By the time IVF is needed, a couple has often experienced a prolonged period of infertility or poor pregnancy outcomes such as multiple miscarriages. Couples who seek IVF because of a genetic condition in the family may have already experienced the loss of a child or other relative. While IVF does provide hope for these couples, the procedure can be time consuming, expensive, and emotionally draining.

Before any of the ARTs are initiated, a series of evaluations occur of both the male and female desiring a pregnancy. These evaluations will help determine the cause of the infertility or any difficulties that may occur in the IVF or PGD process. In addition, both partners are offered genetic testing based on ethnic backgrounds and family histories, such as testing for cystic fibrosis carrier status in Caucasians or sickle cell carrier status in African Americans. For those with a family history of a genetic condition, the specific mutation in the family must be identified before PGD is possible.[2]

There are several ways to perform the IVF process. In some cases, the eggs retrieved will be fertilized in the culture dish. In other cases, the sperm is injected into the egg to increase the fertilization rate. This process is called *intracytoplasmic sperm injection* (ICSI). Depending on the development of the embryos, the laboratory will allow them to grow for either three or five days before deciding which embryos appear to be the healthiest (based on number of cell divisions and visual appearance).[2]

GIFT and ZIFT are variations of IVF. In GIFT, the egg and sperm are retrieved as in IVF, but rather than fertilization occurring in the laboratory the gametes are placed in the woman's fallopian tube with the hope that fertilization will occur in the body. Some couples prefer this method that includes fertilization in the body for religious reasons. In ZIFT, IVF is used and the very early embryo is transferred back to the woman's fallopian tube. Both GIFT and ZIFT are more invasive and costly than IVF. Lastly, in FET, IVF is employed and embryos are frozen for future use. In a future cycle the woman will take medications in pill and injection form to prepare the uterus for the embryo transfer procedure.[2,3]

Success rates of ARTs are reported in a standardized way to the CDC as a live born child rather than an early positive pregnancy test, since this is the information most couples desire. The CDC reports that in 2012, 176,275 ART cycles were performed at 456 reporting clinics in the United States, resulting in 51,294 live births (deliveries of one or more living infants) and 65,179 infants. This is a success rate of 34%, which is improved significantly from 14% in 1989. To understand this number it is helpful to remember that a healthy couple with no fertility problems has about a 20% chance of pregnancy each month. Still, to some, the physical and emotional processes of IVF as well as the high costs (discussed at the end of the chapter) are too burdensome given its 34% success rate. Multiple ART cycles may be needed, which increases financial costs and prolongs the emotional ups and downs.[1]

Benefits and Risks

The benefit of PGD is that a couple can choose to have their own biological child that is free from a genetic condition that runs in the family without having to rely on prenatal diagnosis at 10 weeks gestation or later. By retrieving the egg and sperm and allowing fertilization to occur in the laboratory, testing embryos for disease status and then only transferring embryos without the disease gene, the decision of whether to continue an affected pregnancy is avoided. In fact an affected pregnancy is never started, thus preventing a child from suffering with a genetic condition. However, others believe that creating embryos and then not using them because of their genetic status is unethical and discriminatory. Those who believe that life begins at conception may not find this an acceptable alternative to prenatal diagnosis.

In addition, the IVF procedure comes with some risks. During the process of stimulating multiple eggs to mature, up to 2% of women experience a severe case of ovarian hyperstimulation syndrome in which the ovaries are significantly enlarged, fluid may leak into the abdominal and chest cavities, and may cause difficulty with breathing, blood clots, kidney failure, nausea, diarrhea, and abdominal pain. Most women undergoing IVF have mild symptoms of ovarian hyperstimulation syndrome. If severe symptoms occur, an IVF cycle may be cancelled, symptoms may be treated with medication, or a hospitalization may be required. There has also been a concern that ARTs may be associated with an increased risk for cancer of the breast, ovary, and uterus, although to date there has been no direct correlation between fertility treatments and these cancers. Women with infertility have been shown to have a higher rate of these cancers, but it is not clear that the increase in risk is due to fertility treatments.

A third risk with ARTs includes higher-order pregnancies, since more than one embryo is often transferred to increase the chance of achieving a pregnancy.[2] A higher-order pregnancy is associated with risks that include premature delivery and additional complications related to prematurity. The number of embryos to transfer in a given cycle is a significant question that fertility clinics must address and is discussed in the next section of this chapter. There is also a question as to whether the chances for birth defects or genetic conditions are higher in an IVF pregnancy. The data on this question is difficult to interpret because more IVF pregnancies are higher-order births that come with a higher chance for preterm delivery and associated medical complications. In addition, it is most appropriate to compare babies born after IVF to babies conceived by couples who have experienced infertility, and this data is difficult to obtain. Finally, it is possible that there is an increase in risk for imprinting disorders (in which the particular disorder is only expressed if inherited from the parent of a specific gender), developmental delays, and sex chromosome or other chromosomal aneuploidy. Studies of these possibilities have either been conflicting or shown only a minimal increase in risk compared to non-IVF pregnancies.[2]

History

Like many medical procedures, IVF was first attempted in animals. In 1959 the first rabbit was born after IVF. Human eggs were fertilized in the laboratory in the 1940s, but the first live birth of a child did not occur until 1978 in England when Louis Brown, the first "test tube baby," was born. The development of these procedures, which includes fertilization outside of the body, was controversial. In particular the Catholic Church denounced the practice of IVF in 1949 when Pope Pius XII said that performing IVF was to "take the Lord's work into your own hands." Even within the medical community, some supported the advancement of IVF and others did not. The American Medical Association wanted a halt to IVF research while the American Fertility Society desired to proceed. Research did proceed and Australia was the second country to produce a child born via IVF in 1980, followed soon by the United States in 1981 and France, Sweden and Austria in 1982. Advances in the techniques and methodologies have occurred rapidly since. In 1984 the first baby was born from a frozen embryo as well as a donor egg, while in 1985 the first baby was born to a gestational surrogate after IVF. In 1990 the first pregnancies occurred after PGD. In the 1990s additional advances occurred in assisted hatching of embryos, ICSI, adjustment of medication to help sustain pregnancy once started, modifications of the culture media where fertilization and early embryo growth occur, and improvements in equipment.[4,5]

Number of Embryos to Transfer per *In Vitro* Fertilization Cycle

The issue of the number of embryos to transfer in a given cycle received much publicity in 2009 when Nadya Suleman gave birth to octuplets in California. Ms. Suleman was a single mother living with her parents and already caring for six children, three of whom have disabilities. She used a sperm donor and IVF to become pregnant with her first six children as well as the octuplets. It was later discovered that her physician, Dr. Michael Kamrava, transferred six embryos to Ms. Suleman in one cycle, resulting in eight babies.[6] The Suleman octuplets are the second set of octuplets in the United States that have survived. Higher-order pregnancies are medically difficult because of the chance for premature delivery, which increases proportionately with the number of fetuses. Higher-order gestations likewise more often result in fetal mortality. Even when the babies survive, they may require months of hospitalization and may be affected with conditions associated with prematurity such as vision loss, cerebral palsy, intellectual disabilities, hearing loss, and other conditions.

Fertility clinics desire high success rates with IVF so they can attract more patients. In an attempt to increase success rates, clinics may increase the number of embryos transferred in a given IVF cycle. The American Society for Reproductive Medicine (ASRM) and the Society for Assisted Reproductive Technology (SART) have created guidelines which recommend the number of embryos to transfer in a cycle given the age of the mother, stage of development, and quality of the embryos. The most recent guidelines, published in January of 2013, suggest that for a woman under age 35 the number of embryos that should be transferred in one cycle is one or two.[7] Transferring six, then, is clearly outside of the professional guidelines (Ms. Suleman was 33 years old in 2009).

The ethical principles involved in this case, and any other that could result in a higher-order gestation, are autonomy of the patient and the physician's obligation to beneficence (maximize clinical good) and nonmaleficence (do no harm) for the mother, the pregnancy, and the mother's existing children. The professional guidelines exist so that if a patient were to ask for a higher number embryo transfer than recommended by professional guidelines, the physician's obligations to beneficence and nonmaleficence should clearly limit patient autonomy. The guidelines prevent people who cannot provide true informed consent or demonstrate rational decision-making capacity from receiving a higher-number embryo transfer. For the same reasons of beneficence and nonmaleficence as well as professional integrity, the guidelines are meant to prevent a fertility specialist from offering a higher number embryo transfer.[6]

An additional ethical principle to consider in these situations is that of justice. In particular, there should be consideration of who has access to IVF procedures and the societal burden in resources needed to support children created through higher number embryo transfer who will likely require lengthy hospitalization after birth and may require lifelong medical support. The mother or couple's prior obligations and the possibility of harm to the existing children when seeking a seventh IVF pregnancy, for example, especially one in which six embryos are transferred as in the Suleman case, should be considered. Some fertility specialists may offer women a higher number embryo transfer and then selective reduction to a twin or singleton pregnancy if a higher-order gestation results. However, this may not be a desirable scenario for either the patient (who would have an increased risk for loss of the whole pregnancy with this procedure) or the fertility specialist, who has the dual obligation of beneficence to both the mother and the developing fetuses.[6]

The professional guidelines in the United States are just that—guidelines, not laws. There are no laws in the United States governing the practice of ARTs. The only law is the Fertility Clinic Success Rate and Certification Act of 1992, which requires clinics providing IVF in the United States to report certain data, such as the number of embryos transferred and the success rates. But there is no law dictating how many embryos may be transferred in one cycle.[8] Many other countries, such as the United Kingdom and Canada, have passed legislation regulating the number of embryos to transfer in order to limit the number of higher-order gestations and the complications associated with them. In fact, due to the increases in success rates with ARTs, there is a trend toward single embryo transfer.[9] Still, infractions to the professional guidelines have been punishable, as in the case of Dr. Kamrava. The American Society of Reproductive medicine expelled Dr. Kamrava in 2009, and in 2011 the California Medical Board revoked his medical license.[6]

Gamete Donors and Surrogates

Sometimes in the process of ARTs and for various medical reasons, an outside party is required in order for a couple to have a successful pregnancy. This is also called *collaborative reproduction*. One example is a sperm donor, whose participation is fairly quick and medically risk-free through providing a sperm sample in a donation facility. Another example is an egg donor, whose participation in the process is much more involved and requires the donor to undergo ovarian stimulation. This is a more lengthy process (usually about 6 weeks) requiring the donor to take oral medications, give herself injections, have multiple blood tests and vaginal ultrasounds, and ultimately surgical egg retrieval. Another example of collaborative reproduction is surrogacy. A traditional surrogate donates her eggs as well as her uterus in carrying a pregnancy. A gestational surrogate or carrier, as the name implies, carries the pregnancy for another couple who has undergone IVF with their own egg and sperm. Gestational surrogacy is the most commonly used form of surrogacy.[8,10]

Financial Compensation

The ASRM encourages financial compensation for both egg and sperm donors. However, they acknowledge that this raises ethical questions particularly for egg donors, such as whether recruitment strategies that include financial compensation protect the interests of the egg donor or devalue human life by treating human eggs as commodities. In their Ethics Committee Opinion on this subject, the ASRM designates that the financial compensation is for the "time, inconvenience and discomfort" (p. 306) associated with egg or sperm retrieval, not for the gametes themselves.[11] The ASRM recommends financial compensation of approximately $5000 for egg donors and, in general, fertility clinics tend to follow these guidelines. Private individuals or companies may not. They may advertise for an egg donor with specific characteristics such as a high intelligence quotient, specific hair color, musical ability, or other abilities and be willing to pay a higher price for them. Advertisements for egg donors often occur on the Internet or in college newspapers. Women in financial need may discount medical and psychological risks associated with egg donation. A college student in need of money to pay tuition might sign away her legal rights to eggs she donates at age 18, but find herself distraught by the fact that she may have a biological child that she does not know at age 30. The financial need may be so great that some women might be willing to hide some of their medical information so that they appear to be good egg donors. Additionally, paying high prices for specific qualities in egg donors may be seen as a form of positive eugenics, accessible only to those with financial means.[11]

In response to these concerns, the ASRM recommends that fertility centers provide detailed counseling to prospective egg and sperm donors regarding possible medical and psychological risks of donation. They also recommend that donors consider how they may feel in the future about their current decision to donate, and they recommend that donors be over age 21. Further, they recommend that clinics try to assess whether a woman feels coerced into her decision based on her financial situation. They recommend that advertisements for donors be accurate and responsible and, in order to limit the health risks to a donor, they recommend limiting the number of times an individual may donate. Although there are laws in the United States prohibiting financial compensation of organ donors, no laws currently exist to regulate the compensation of gamete donors.[11]

Financial compensation for surrogates is greater than for egg or sperm donors, considering the length of time involved in carrying a pregnancy and the physical exertion of the birth process. Compensation typically covers the costs associated with prenatal care and delivery. In 2008 in the United States, the average payment to a surrogate was $20,000. As with egg donors, there is the potential for exploitation of surrogates.[8]

Medical and Psychological Risks

Medical risks with gamete donation primarily relate to egg donors, since sperm donation is a brief and noninvasive process.

Egg donors, however, have the risks of the fertility medications (which include the possibility of ovarian hyperstimulation syndrome described earlier) and the surgical risks associated with the egg retrieval process. The ASRM recommends that fertility clinics ensure that egg donors understand these medical risks through a detailed informed consent process and have health insurance that covers any complications that arise from these procedures before initiating the egg donation process. In addition, most fertility centers require donors to undergo genetic screening based on their ethnic background and family history. These tests may reveal information that will affect the donor's health or the health of her future offspring. A donor should be informed of these tests and decide whether she is ready to procure this knowledge. Surrogates should be informed of the medical risks associated with carrying and delivering a baby.[8,11]

Whether donors have the right to know the outcomes of their donations or to place limitations on their donations are further ethical issues to consider. Some donors prefer to know if a pregnancy or child ever results from the donation for various reasons, including that they may know that future contact is possible. The donor may also desire medical information about the health of any child that results to inform his or her own future reproductive attempts. Donors may also wish to place limitations on their donations. For instance, some donors may like to designate that their gametes go to a couple under age 40, or only male–female couples, or only Caucasians. Currently, clinics have differing policies on these issues. The Ethics Committee of the ASRM encourages informing donors about any children born and their health, but discourages limitations on donor gametes based on donor preferences. The ASRM also encourages donors to consider how their choices to donate gametes may affect their relationships in the future. They may wish to consider how future spouses may feel about them already having biological children and how future children may feel about having biological half-siblings.[12]

Surrogacy has its own set of psychological risks of harm that potential surrogates should be encouraged to explore and consider as part of the informed consent process. Some women may find it very difficult to surrender a child after carrying it for 40 weeks and to potentially have no further contact. Women may change their minds about keeping a child after signing a contract with a couple to do so. There have been cases in the United States where surrogates have changed their minds and courts upheld their rights to keep the children they carried, even if they were not genetically related to the child.[8]

Donor Right to Anonymity versus Rights of Offspring Conceived

Currently, fertility and donation centers have a variety of policies regarding contact and information sharing between donors and offspring. This variety reflects the ongoing debate over whose rights are more important. Is it more important for a donor to have the right to remain anonymous, which is the preference of most donors and therefore increases the number of donors? Or is the right of the offspring to know his or her biological parent more important? Offspring of donors may wish to have medical information about the donor that may not have been collected at the time of the donation or has occurred after the donation. Family medical history is an important way that individuals become aware of conditions they may be at risk for in the future and for which they may be able to be monitored for symptoms or participate in preventative behaviors if they know of the increased risk. The ASRM encourages fertility centers to require or encourage donors to share updated medical information over time, whether it is an anonymous fashion or not.[13] Additionally, it appears that many offspring would like to know more about their donor or biological half-siblings as evidenced by the creation of the website The Donor Sibling Registry. This is a website where individuals who have been conceived through gamete donation can go to search for their donors or half-siblings. The site currently has 41,000 paying registrants who are primarily donors or individuals conceived by donors.[14]

The Ethics Committee of the ASRM encourages the disclosure to offspring of their conception by gamete donation.[13] They have identified four levels of information sharing that donors may be offered. The levels ranges from complete anonymity with no personally identifying information shared to a donor agreeing to share personally identifying information if the offspring requests it at the age of maturity. Options in between these include sharing updated medical information with the donation center in a nonidentifying manner and the donor agreeing to nonidentifying contact through the donation center if requested by the child at the age of maturity. The ASRM encourages fertility and donation centers to have flexible policies that reflect the various preferences of donors, recipients, and offspring.[13] Donors should be made aware of the policy of a particular clinic before donation to ensure that the policy is in line with their desires regarding anonymity and gamete donation. It is also important for donors to be aware that laws and fertility clinic or donation center policies regarding anonymity may change over time and that anonymity cannot be guaranteed. This risk to privacy may affect whether someone is willing to be a donor.[12]

Family Members as Donors or Surrogates

There are a number of reasons a couple may choose to use a family member as a donor. These reasons include that the child would still be biologically related to one of the parents, the family members may desire to help the couple, and relatives may be willing to provide the donation at no financial cost. An ethical issue regarding related donors is whether the donor can make a free and autonomous decision to participate. A relative may feel obligated or pressured to donate, and there could be relational distancing if they decline to donate. For example, a mother who divorces and remarries may expect her grown daughter to donate her eggs or be a surrogate for her. The daughter may feel obligated to do so, especially if she is still a dependent of the mother. Another ethical issue is the confusion that can arise in familial roles when an aunt, for instance, is the biological mother. Is she able to maintain her role as aunt and allow her sister to mother the child, or might she become over-involved with the child to the point where her sister feels uncomfortable? Or maybe the aunt feels like the sister "owes" her and expects special favors and rewards indefinitely. A third issue that arises is how the relative will be viewed in the family if the donation is not successful. Will he or she be blamed? Will others in the family be disappointed or angry with the donor? What if a child results but has a genetic condition or birth defect? Will that be seen as the fault of the donor?

A fourth concern involves the partner of the donor relative. What if his or her expectations of the donor are in conflict with those of the rest of the family? The donor may be caught in the middle of family tensions. A fifth issue is when and how to disclose to a child that a relative he or she likely knows is his or her biological parent. Will this been seen by the offspring as a family secret that should have been revealed earlier? Will he or she feel duped? The Ethics Committee of the ASRM recognizes the rights of families to participate in certain types of collaborative reproduction. They discourage any type of donation that would be consanguineous or incestuous if it occurred through sexual intercourse. The ASRM strongly recommends psychological counseling for families considering intrafamilial donation and detailed informed consent to include a careful review of whether a family member feels coerced to donate. In addition, legal relationships among the parties involved should be clearly documented.[10]

Preimplantation Genetic Diagnosis

Preimplantation Genetic Diagnosis (PGD) is a method of performing genetic testing before a pregnancy starts to determine if a particular genetic condition is present. People who might consider the use of PGD include those who wish to test or screen embryos for an unusual chromosome number, such as women over age 35; carriers of a balanced chromosome translocation that can result in an unbalanced rearrangement in a child; and individuals or couples at risk of passing on a single gene disorder to a child, such as when a parent is affected with an autosomal dominant or X-linked condition or both parents are carriers of an autosomal recessive condition.

PGD can be performed in three ways. First, eggs that are retrieved during an IVF cycle can be tested for a genetic condition by a process of exclusion. The first polar body, or immature egg cell produced at the same time as the mature egg cell, can be tested and if it does contain the genetic mutation then the mature egg should not. Fertilization occurs, and then the second polar body is tested to be sure it does not contain the mutation, confirming the status of the mature egg, which should be the same. This method can be used to test for maternally inherited mutations only, not paternally inherited mutations. The second PGD method is called a *blastomere biopsy* and involves IVF followed by an embryo biopsy at day three after fertilization. At this stage, the cells of the embryo are called *blastomeres*, with six to eight cells present in the embryo. One cell from the embryo is removed for genetic testing. If the embryo is free of the mutation, it could be chosen for transfer to the mother. One problem with this method is that in this early stage of development, embryos can have a mixture of cells, some with the usual number of chromosomes and some with more or less than the usual 46 chromosomes. This phenomenon of mosaicism can give an incorrect result. For example, it may be that the cell that is biopsied has the normal number of chromosomes but the rest of the cells have an extra chromosome, therefore resulting in a child who would most likely be affected with the condition. The third method for PGD is called a *blastocyst biopsy*. In this case, the embryo is biopsied on day five or six when more cells compose the embryo. A few cells can be removed and tested for a genetic mutation. Mosaicism is less common at this stage of development. Embryos would be frozen after a blastocyst biopsy but available for future IVF cycles. Follow-up prenatal genetic diagnosis is recommended during pregnancies conceived with IVF and PGD, although the chances for errors in the PGD process are small.[15]

All three methods used in PGD involve the creation of embryos that are tested and then most often discarded if they have the particular mutation or chromosomal rearrangement in the family. In PGD, affected embryos are not usually transferred to a woman's uterus where they can implant and therefore are not considered a pregnancy. However, some have moral or ethical dilemmas with these technologies because they involve the creation and possible discarding of embryos that have the potential to become human beings if transferred to a woman. In the United States there are currently no federal or state regulations regarding the uses of PGD. In addition, there are currently no professional guidelines to assist clinicians with acceptable uses of the technology. There has been one study in the United States that indicated that directors of fertility clinics are interested in the development of professional guidelines with regard to PGD, but this has not occurred yet.[16] Other countries have either banned PGD (Germany, Switzerland, Austria, Ireland), or have federal regulations that require a license for each new genetic test that is offered by a clinic (United Kingdom, Canada), or have professional guidelines (Japan). The freedom to offer a wider variety of genetic tests in the United States has led to the fact that two-thirds of the world's fertility clinics can be found here. There is substantial international commerce for PGD with foreigners traveling to the United States for the services they desire.[17]

Adult-Onset Disorders

While the first uses of PGD were for the most serious or fatal genetic conditions, they have since expanded. Some clinics offer genetic testing for a late-onset disorder called Huntington disease, a progressive neurologic disease with symptoms that begin at age 35–40 years. Individuals with Huntington disease have several decades of potentially healthy living before the onset of a serious condition. Some believe that PGD should not be used in such instances, while others feel the uses of PGD should be left to those seeking the services. The desire of the individual who may have seen a relative live and die with Huntington disease or has been diagnosed with the condition and wishes to avoid the birth of a child with the condition is compelling. Critics argue that since an individual with a serious late-onset disorder will not be able to care for the child he or she wishes to create, the autonomy of that individual should be limited.

Others suggest that PGD for late-onset disorders should only be offered if the penetrance or chance of being symptomatic for the condition is complete, as in the case of Huntington disease. Recently, the United Kingdom issued a license for testing for the BRCA1 and 2 genes through PGD. Critics of this policy suggest that since the chance of having breast or ovarian cancer even if one inherits a mutation in one of these genes is not 100%, embryos should not be created and discarded based on having a mutation. Proponents state that PGD is warranted because these cancers are life-threatening. Critics also argue that for late-onset conditions, the chance for improvements in future treatments or cures precludes PGD. Others recommend considering the likely age of onset or life expectancy of particular conditions as ways of determining which conditions are appropriate for PGD. However, any lines drawn are somewhat arbitrary. Can a condition with age of onset of 45 not be eligible for PGD, while one with age of onset of 50 is eligible? Or, can life expectancy of age 50 with current treatments mean a condition is eligible for

PGD but not a condition with life expectancy of age 55? Who is to decide whether those lives were worth living or there was enough time for an individual to have a positive life experience? Who determines what amount of suffering is too much? There are those who wish to prevent a "wrongful life," one that would have been better not to exist at all. Disabilities rights activists would counter that the disability is not the problem but rather the society that does not accept and properly accommodate those with disabilities. Further, expanding the uses of PGD raises the specter of eugenics. Should there be a line that will not be crossed in order to prevent the abuses of the past?[18,19]

Consider the family depicted in our clinical scenario in which the patriarch John has early-onset Alzheimer disease. His daughter Amy is 28 years old and pregnant. She is not sure she wishes to be tested, but she desires testing for her son and current pregnancy. While not utilized during her two pregnancies, one option for Amy in the future if she desires another child would be nondisclosing PGD. In other words, she could go through IVF and PGD and only have unaffected embryos transferred as is usually the case. The laboratory would not disclose whether she or any of the other embryos have the mutation in the family, but would just transfer the unaffected embryos. Amy would need thorough informed consent reviewing the ethical issues described above before proceeding on this path.

Preimplantation Genetic Diagnosis for Nonmedical Traits

While using PGD for late-onset disorders is controversial, the use of PGD for nonmedical purposes is even more so. Currently, worldwide the most widely sought nonmedical trait for PGD is gender. Arguments against selection of the gender of the first child primarily revolve around discrimination and stigmatization of the less chosen gender. In countries where typically the male gender is preferred, the practice of PGD for male gender would further the already occurring discrimination and stigmatization of females. It also leads to a skewing of the male to female gender ratio, which can be problematic for males who desire to find female partners of the same nationality. Proponents argue that allowing PGD for gender selection would decrease the practice of ultrasound and abortion if the fetus is of the less desired gender.[20,21]

In the United States, more often gender selection is desired for family balancing. A couple may have one or more children of one gender and desire the next child to be of the opposite gender. The ethical question is whether the desire of parents for family balancing warrants the creation and then discarding of embryos of the undesired gender. Proponents uphold the rights and autonomy of the parents to make such reproductive decisions. Critics are concerned about the slippery slope (PGD for intelligence, strength, beauty) and agree that there should be a public policy that governs such decisions rather than leaving it in the hands of parents. They question whether gender selection is the best use of a limited medical resource and whether a child chosen for its gender may undergo psychological harms if he or she does not live up to gender stereotypes.[20,21] In 1999 the Ethics Committee of the ASRM published an opinion that PGD should not be used solely for gender selection.[21] It also published a statement in 2001 that supported gender selection through preconception sperm sorting and then intrauterine insemination using sperm more likely to carry the chromosome of choice for gender. Although less accurate, this is a much less invasive and costly process than PGD and does not involve the creation of embryos outside the body. They did recommend certain practices for couples seeking preconception gender selection, such as informing them of the risk of failure, asking them to affirm that they will accept a child of the less desired gender, counseling them regarding unrealistic expectations of a child of the desired gender, and encouraging them to participate in research on this topic so that it can be better understood in the future.[22]

Creating a Donor Sibling

A further extension of PGD is to select a trait that has no medical benefit to the offspring being created but is chosen to help a family member. One example is using IVF and PGD to select an embryo that is an HLA match for a sibling who needs a stem cell transplant. An increasing number of medical conditions are treated with stem cell therapy. A well-publicized case of this use of PGD occurred in 2000 when the Nash family gave birth to their son Adam, who was created to be a stem cell donor for his sister Molly. Molly had a genetic condition called *Fanconi anemia*, an autosomal recessive condition. She had the usual features of FA including fused joints, a missing thumb, incomplete development of the gut, and, ultimately, leukemia. In order to cure Molly's leukemia, a stem cell transplant from someone who was an HLA match was needed. Molly's parents decided to use IVF and PGD, first to ensure that their next child did not have FA and second to ensure that this child would be an HLA match for Molly. Adam resulted from the embryo that fit both criteria. After birth, the stem cells from his umbilical cord were collected and given to Molly. Molly was cured of leukemia, although she still has FA.[23]

In the Nash case, Adam was tested for FA as well as a nonmedical trait. The case brings up the possibility that others may choose only to test for the nonmedical trait. And if couples are permitted to test for HLA status, what comes next? Does this lead the way to PGD for enhancement rather than to prevent a disease? As with PGD for late-onset disorders, PGD for nonmedical traits invokes fears of eugenics. By selecting enhancements, people may select against those without them. Is it possible to follow the path of reproductive freedoms to this extent, or will the abuses of the past reoccur? Will the practice of creating sibling donors commodity children for their parts? In the case of the Nash family, they welcomed Adam into the family—but what if another family did the same but chose to put their donor child up for adoption after collecting the stem cells? Or what if a family created a donor sibling but then had an abortion, at which time stem cells were collected? Would those uses of the technology be permissible or desirable? And what are the donor sibling's obligations throughout his or her lifetime? For instance, sometimes children with FA need kidney transplants. Will Adam be expected by his family to donate a kidney if that scenario arises?[23]

Other issues regarding donor siblings are the costs and burdens of PGD. The Nash family spent over $100,000 for five IVF and PGD attempts before a successful pregnancy with Adam. There was no insurance coverage and they paid out of pocket. The Nashes admit that they were very fortunate to have the financial means to create Adam. Many others in the same situation would not have the financial means. Thus, the issue surfaces of justice and access to this form of treatment available to only a few. In the process of creating Adam the Nashes created over 25 other embryos that are still frozen. The ethical issue of the fate of all those frozen embryos and whether they should have been created arises once again.[23]

Selecting for a Disability

People with certain disabilities live in communities in which having the disability is important to being a true member of the community. Examples of these are the deaf and the short stature (dwarfism) communities. With the possibilities available now through PGD, some parents with these traits have requested PGD to ensure that their child will have the disability in the family and community. It is generally agreed that parents have duties and obligations toward their children to give them the best possible lives and opportunities. But in the context of a different social community, what is best may be subjective. The reproductive rights of the parents are juxtaposed with the best interests of the child. Consider the example of hearing. Most would agree that hearing is better than not hearing. A person's experiences (to hear voices and music) and opportunities (for work, school, and relationships) are broadened by the ability to hear. A hearing person will not experience discrimination and the need for accommodation that a nonhearing person may. Yet within their community, deafness is the key to admittance. That is certainly not to say that a deaf person cannot have a full and meaningful life. But, all other things being equal, hearing is valuable to a human being. This raises the question of who really benefits from the creation of a deaf child. If both parents are deaf and have a strong deaf community, then the parents certainly benefit. Parents may also find it easier to communicate and bond with a deaf child. Proponents of allowing parents to select for deafness argue that nothing was taken away from the child if the child could never hear, and that the creation of the child who cannot hear is better than that child never existing. They also argue that others cannot determine what should be considered a "good" life. Critics argue that no matter what benefits may come from being accepted into the deaf community, they do not outweigh the benefits of being able to hear in a world that is mostly hearing. Some critics advocate for legislation or guidelines in the United States that would prevent the use of PGD for selecting embryos with disabilities.[24]

Microarrays and Preimplantation Genetic Diagnosis

In some cases PGD is performed to determine if aneuploidy, or a change in the chromosome number from the usual 46 chromosomes, is present in an embryo. Typically this is done through a technique called *fluorescence in situ hybridization* (FISH), in which a fluorescent probe that binds to the centromeres of the chromosomes most often involved in aneuploidy is used. More recently, a newer technique called *chromosome microarray* (CMA) testing is being used instead. The advantage of this technology is that it can detect not only aneuploidy but also large and small unbalanced structural abnormalities and uniparental disomy (inheriting both copies of a gene from one parent rather than each parent contributing a copy), if an array that detects changes in single nucleotides (SNP array) is used. Using CMA allows for a broad detection of genetic changes that could be clinically significant for a child. However, a problem with the use of CMAs is the interpretation of submicroscopic chromosomal imbalances that are detected. Many of these are benign copy number variants with no clinical significance, while others may cause birth defects and mental retardation. Data is being collected to help determine which imbalances are likely to be clinically significant, but at this time it is difficult to interpret some of the findings from CMA testing. It is not clear whether embryos with imbalances of unclear significance would be chosen for transfer. It is likely that if there were other embryos available at the time, the ones with variants of unknown significance would not be chosen. In some cases the embryo(s) with the variant may be the only one(s) left. How clinics handle the disclosure and counseling regarding this information is yet to be determined, since CMA use in PGD is still in the research stage.[25]

Preserving Fertility

With advances in the ability to freeze sperm, oocytes, and embryos, the possibility of delaying reproduction for various reasons exists. The uses of ARTs in preserving fertility for various reasons are discussed below.

How Old is Too Old?

The oldest woman to give birth as of 2008 was a 70-year-old woman in India who had a long history of infertility. The pregnancy was achieved with the use of a donor egg and her husband's sperm, although the 70-year-old woman carried and gave birth herself with the help of hormones to support the pregnancy since she was postmenopausal.[26] This couple raises the question of how old is too old to have a baby. If the parents are likely to die of natural causes before the child reaches age 18, is that too old? This was the case for a single woman in Spain who gave birth to twins at the age of 66 using donor egg and sperm. She died three years later of cancer, leaving her children as orphans.[27] Is it selfish of older parents to create lives when they will not likely be alive to financially or emotionally support the children? Or what about cases where one parent is much older, but the other would likely still survive to raise the child? Some fertility clinics have an age limit, such as age 55, due to health risks for older mothers and babies. After this age they recommend a gestational surrogate.[28]

Some argue that an individual's autonomy should prevail, and that the suffering of the childless should allow for reproduction at any age. However, IVF services and donor eggs are a limited service. Should priority be given to older women? Or perhaps priority should be given only if they have never had children? The desperation of some older women to have a child at a later age has led to women lying about age to get IVF services.[29] As for premenopausal women who can still conceive but may be over age 45, the risk for aneuploidy increases significantly as do the chances for complications for mother and baby. For now in the United States, individual clinics determine their own age cut-offs.

Children and Teens with Cancer or Other Chronic Illnesses

With the technology now to cryopreserve sperm, embryos and oocytes, there are new opportunities for people to preserve fertility when there is a threat to future reproduction. One instance of this is cancer patients whose treatment will likely make them infertile or damage reproductive organs or gametes. If cancer is diagnosed in an adult before he or she has reproduced, the ASRM recommends that the oncologist discuss ways to obtain and cryopreserve gametes if the person is single, or embryos if he or she has a partner. For postpubertal males, providing a sperm sample is all that is needed. For prepubertal males, sperm can be removed from the testes with a needle. Postpubertal females can go through ovarian stimulation and egg retrieval as with a usual IVF cycle. The oncologist, in the case of postpubertal females with cancer, should inform patients and their families about the possible risks of delaying cancer treatment in order to pursue techniques to preserve fertility and how the hormones involved in those techniques may affect the cancer. Prepubertal females can have ovarian tissue removed laparoscopically and cryopreserved.[30,31]

The issue becomes more difficult when the cancer diagnosis is made in a child or adolescent. Then questions arise as to who can give informed consent for procedures to obtain gametes. The Ethics and Practice Committees of the ASRM recommend that parents can give consent if and only if the minor agrees to the procedures. The reasoning for allowing parental consent is that the procedures are likely to benefit the child in the future. However, children may not be able to understand the future benefit and may not wish to undergo procedures in addition to those to treat their cancer. There are also questions about whether a person who has been diagnosed with more serious forms of cancer should be offered the same options for fertility preservation, given that it is not likely he or she will survive to raise a child. However, many children have lost a parent and have had meaningful lives. It may be argued that a single person with cancer should be restricted from using IVF with a donor egg or sperm, since if he or she died from a recurrence, perhaps triggered by IVF hormones, there would not be a second parent to raise the child. Additionally, fertility clinics are encouraged to seek directives from individuals or their parents choosing to preserve fertility so that if they do die from their cancer it is clear what should be done with any stored gametes or embryos or who should be able to decide. In the event a person has an inherited form of cancer, the option of IVF and PGD to ensure the offspring will not inherit the mutation is considered acceptable in the United States.[30]

Individuals with certain genetic conditions may also wish to use fertility preservation. Females with Turner syndrome or who carry the Fragile X syndrome premutation could have oocyte or ovarian tissue cryopreservation while they are young, since premature ovarian failure is likely to occur. While it is not recommended for routine practice by the ASRM yet, it is also possible that young healthy women who wish to delay childbearing could have oocyte or ovarian tissue cryopreservation so that by the time they are ready to reproduce, their eggs are still young and the chance for aneuploidy has not increased. Given the costs involved, this could create a question of access and justice where those with means can have healthier children than those without.[31]

Posthumous Reproduction

Upon the death of an individual who has chosen to store gametes or embryos, a surviving spouse, partner, or other family member may chose to use the stored materials to create a child. In these instances, fertility clinics most likely have requested that individuals indicate their wishes for their gametes or embryos after their death. These wishes usually dictate whether requests from family members to use the samples will be permitted. Alternatively, the spouse of a person in a persistent vegetative state or who is brain dead or very recently deceased may request sperm or oocyte retrieval. These situations more often arise due to accidents, and the individual from whom gametes are requested most likely did not indicate whether he or she would have wanted gametes used under these circumstances.[32] In 2000, Strong, Gingrich, and

Kutteh reported on a case in which they were asked to retrieve sperm from a 31-year-old male with a history of heart problems who had a sudden cardiac arrest and deteriorated to the point where he was on a respirator and physicians felt it was unlikely he could recover. The family agreed to extubation, but his wife of two months inquired about the possibility of sperm retrieval before death. Family members on both sides felt that the man would have liked to have had children in the usual course of his marriage and life, and no one objected to the request. The ethical question was whether family members may have been biased. The physicians brought the case to their hospital ethics committee, who gave mainly legal advice but were unable to address the ethical issues of conceiving a child after or just preceding the death of a parent. In these cases, physicians look to the family members to determine if inferred consent can be obtained. Did the individual ever express to anyone in the family what he or she would have wanted in such a case? If not, requests for use of gametes or embryos may be denied.[33]

The legal and social status of children conceived after the death of a parent is unclear. Are children conceived after the death of a parent the legal heirs of that parent? Do they have rights to the inheritance left behind by the deceased parent? Once again, different countries have different laws about whether the practice of posthumous reproduction is permitted and, if so, in what circumstances and with what benefits. The Ethics Committee of the ASRM opines that the wishes of the donor, if made known, should not be overruled by the desires of family members. They also state that in situations where embryos were stored and then a wife dies, care should be taken in cases where the husband remarries and then wishes to use the embryos from his first marriage to create a child with his second wife. Every effort should be made by fertility clinics to ensure that the second wife, who is now the surrogate, is not being unduly pressured or that her welfare is not in jeopardy. The advent of gamete and embryo freezing has allowed circumstances to arise that raise ethical questions regarding posthumous reproduction. Clinics should carefully consider these questions.[32]

Cloning

Also known as *somatic cell nuclear transfer* (SCNT), cloning is the process of taking a somatic cell from one organism and transferring it to the oocyte of another whose genetic material has been removed. Thus, the somatic cell is diploid and the entire genome of the first organism is being replicated. Many are familiar with the 1997 story of the first cloned lamb named Dolly. So far, it appears the process of SCNT is not very efficient and leads to offspring with an increase in birth defects and early aging. The safety and efficacy issues of this technique have yet to be determined. Still, many have taken sides as to whether the process is ethical. On the side of SCNT as ethical, proponents state the advantage of SCNT to help infertile couples conceive a child who is genetically related (in this case identical) to one of the parents. Infertile couples may prefer this to using an anonymous donor. Second, proponents point to the possibility of avoiding genetic conditions, such as those inherited in autosomal recessive or dominant patterns, by using the genome of only one unaffected parent. Of course ARTs can currently achieve the same goals by other means. On the side of SCNT as unethical, critics point to the fact that for the first time new human beings could be created without the joining of two genomes. This may devalue the genetic individuality of humans and, if used on a wide spread basis, could restrict genetic diversity. The child clone would still have unique experiences, upbringing, education, and different mitochondrial DNA from the mother, leading to some individuality. There is the concern that the creation of such a child may serve the needs of one or both parents but may not be in the best interests of the child. In fact, SCNT may be considered experimentation on the child. The child may be subject to unreasonable expectations that he or she look or behave like the parent. Parents may be disappointed, for instance, if they use cells from a deceased child to create his/her clone and the clone is not identical. SCNT may also be another way that single people choose to have a child, making two-parent homes less common. Last, there may be the creation of a new market for genome donors for SCNT which could take society down the path of eugenics once again, where people with means are able to choose the traits of their children. The Ethics Committee of the ASRM suggests that caution be used with any future clinical application of SCNT since there is so much skepticism in the public. The ASRM states that currently SCNT does not meet the standard for being ethically acceptable but that research using SCNT is not prohibited if performed in an ethical manner.[34]

Fate of Frozen Embryos

Another area of ethical debate in ARTs is the fate of the frozen embryos. As described earlier, often more embryos are created than used in the treatment of infertility or when PGD is performed. How one may view this question may depend on how one sees the status of the human embryo, as is the case for many of the issues related to ARTs. If one perceives the embryo to have the same rights as a person, since the embryo has the potential to become a human being if transferred to a uterus, then one is likely to choose different options for extra embryos than if one sees the embryo as special but not deserving all the rights of a person. The most conservative view may conclude that extra embryos should not be created at all, namely that IVF should only be used to retrieve one or two eggs at a time so that extra embryos are not created. Currently there are over 500,000 embryos in the United States in indefinite frozen storage. For those who hold that embryos should have the same rights as people, this land of limbo is not acceptable. Some couples are actively in the process of using those frozen embryos in their own IVF cycles. For these couples there is no intent to keep the embryos frozen indefinitely. Once a couple has completed its family, there is a choice about what to do with any remaining embryos. One option is to donate the embryos to another infertile couple so that they can achieve a pregnancy. The problem with this option is that there are far more frozen embryos than infertile couples looking for embryos. Only a small fraction of those frozen can be used in this way.[35]

Another option couples have is to donate their embryos to research such as stem cell research. Embryos are a source of stem cells that can become many cell types in the body, making them a good source for potential treatments or cures for diseases. Embryonic stem cell research is controversial, although legal in the United States. The Ethics Committee of the ASRM endorses the use of embryos for stem cell research. Their position is due in part to the fact that if discarded the embryos would serve no purpose, but if they are donated to embryonic stem cell research they may further the discovery of treatments or cures for illnesses such as Parkinson and Alzheimer diseases. Critics argue that the practice of using embryos that remain after ARTs will lead to the creation of embryos for the purpose of treating or curing diseases. The ASRM does state that embryos should not be bought or sold.

Thus, two options remain. Some couples choose to have the embryo transferred to the uterus but at a time in the menstrual cycle when the woman is less likely to conceive. They may see this as a more natural process than any of the remaining options. The last option is to permit the fertility clinic to thaw the embryos and dispose of them. Currently the ASRM recommends that couples be made aware of these options and asked to indicate a preference in case something should happen to them and they are no longer able to indicate their wishes for the embryos.

Access

There are a number of reasons that there is not equal access to ARTs in the United States and other countries. The first of these is cost. The average cost in the United States for one IVF cycle is about $10,000. Often more than one cycle is needed to have a child. In addition, there is no insurance coverage for ARTs in the United States, although a few states may cover some expenses. One way to make the distribution of ARTs more equitable would be for all states or the federal government to provide insurance coverage to infertile couples. However, even in countries with socialized medicine, such as the United Kingdom, the long wait for services causes couples to seek private clinics and pay out of pocket.[8]

Fertility clinics may also have policies about who they will serve. For instance, they may choose to serve only married couples under age 45. In particular, they may exclude single people desiring to have a child or gay and lesbian individuals or couples. The Ethics Committee of the ASRM states that fertility clinics should provide services for individuals or couples regardless of their marriage status or sexual orientation.[36]

Summary

Many of the ethical issues surrounding ARTs pertain to the autonomy of the individual as compared to obligations of physicians for beneficence and nonmaleficence. The right to privacy for gamete donors and surrogates competes with the desire of some offspring of donors to know their biological parents. The risks for coercion of donors and surrogates through financial compensation and the commodification of gametes are ethical questions that warrant further consideration. Acceptable uses of IVF and PGD need further public discourse. The justice of creating a child when one or both parents is/are either deceased or older deserves attention. Underlying all these questions is perhaps the primary question regarding the moral status of the embryo and how that status should dictate usage. Should the United States be a nation where individuals have total reproductive freedom, or should there be limits? Does the history of eugenics in the United States warrant limitations in order to prevent abuses? Will unequal access to IVF and PGD services translate into two classes of society, one of which will have access to improved health and enhancements because they can afford them? Will professional guidelines be enough to navigate these muddy waters, or will there be a need for legislation? Currently, fertility clinics in the United States have a wide open playing field with little oversight.

REFERENCES

1. Centers for Disease Control and Prevention. (2012). Assisted Reproductive Technology. Available at: http://www.cdc.gov/art/. Accessed January 15, 2013.
2. Society for Assisted Reproductive Technologies. (1996–2013). Assisted reproductive technologies. Available at: http://www.sart.org/SART_Assisted_Reproductive_Technologies/. Accessed January 15, 2013.
3. Resolve: The National Fertility Association. (2013). IVF/ART. Available at: http://www.resolve.org/family-building-options/ivf-art.html. Accessed January 15, 2013.
4. Public Broadcasting Service. (1996–2010). *The American Experience: 25 Years*. Timeline: The History of In Vitro Fertilization. Available at: http://www.pbs.org/wgbh/americanexperience/features/timeline/babies/. Accessed January 15, 2013.
5. IVF Worldwide. (2012). IVF history. Available at: http://www.ivf-worldwide.com/ivf-history.html. Accessed January 15, 2013.
6. Rosenthal, M.S. (2010). The Suleman octuplet case: an analysis of multiple ethical issues. *Women's Health Issues*. 20(4):260–265.
7. The Practice Committee of the American Society for Reproductive Medicine and the Practice Committee of the Society for

Reproductive Technology. (2013). Criteria for number of embryos to transfer: a committee opinion. *Fertility and Sterility.* 99(1):44–46.

8. Brezina, P.R., Zhao, Y. (2012). The ethical, legal, and social issues impacted by modern assisted reproductive technologies. *Obstetrics and Gynecology International.* 1–7.
9. Practice Committee of the Society for Assisted Reproductive Technology and Practice Committee of the American Society for Reproductive Medicine. (2012). Elective single-embryo transfer. *Fertility and Sterility.* 97(4):835–842.
10. The Ethics Committee of the American Society of Reproductive Medicine. (2012). Using family members as gamete donors or surrogates. *Fertility and Sterility.* 98(4):797–803.
11. The Ethics Committee of the American Society for Reproductive Medicine. (2007). Financial compensation of oocyte donors. *Fertility and Sterility.* 88(2):305–309.
12. Ethics Society of the American Society for Reproductive Medicine. (2009). Interests, obligations, and rights of the donor in gamete donation. *Fertility and Sterility.* 91(1):22–27.
13. Ethics Committee of the American Society for Reproductive Medicine. (2004). Informing offspring of their conception by gamete donation. *Fertility and Sterility.* 81(3):527–531.
14. The Donor Sibling Registry: Educating, Connecting and Supporting Donor Families. Available at: https://www.donorsiblingregistry.com/. Accessed June 12, 2014.
15. Reproductive Genetics Institute. (2013). Preimplantation genetic diagnosis. Available at: http://reproductivegenetics.com/preimplantation-genetic-diagnosis-pgd-faq/. Accessed January 22, 2013.
16. Baruch, S., Kaufman, D., Hudson, K.L. (2008). Genetic testing of embryos: practices and perspectives of US in vitro fertilization clinics. *Fertility and Sterility.* 89 (5):1053–1058.
17. The Savior Siblings Blog. (2009). Is PGD being regulated? Available at: http://ourethicaljourney09.blogspot.com/2009/06/is-big-brother-watching-pgd-regulations.html. Accessed January 22, 2013.
18. Krahn, T. (2009). Preimplantation genetic diagnosis: does age of onset matter (anymore)? *Medicine, Health Care, and Philosophy.* 12(2):187–202.

19. Noble, R., Bahadur, G., Iqbal, M., Sanyal, A. (2008). Pandora's Box: ethics of PGD for inherited risk of late-onset disorders. *Reproductive Biomedicine Online*. 17(3):55–60.
20. Robertson, J.A. (2003). Extending preimplantation genetic diagnosis: medical and non-medical uses. *Journal of Medical Ethics*. 29:213–216.
21. The Ethics Committee of the American Society for Reproductive Medicine. (1999). Sex selection and preimplantation genetic diagnosis. *Fertility and Sterility*. (72)4:595–598.
22. The Ethics Committee of the American Society for Reproductive Medicine. (2001). Preconception gender selection for nonmedical reasons. *Fertility and Sterility*. (75)5:861–864.
23. Kahn, J.P. and Mastroianni, A.C. (2004). Creating a stem cell donor: a case study in reproductive genetics. *Kennedy Institute of Ethics Journal*. (14)1:81–96.
24. Murphy, T.F. (2009). Choosing disabilities and enhancements in children: a choice too far? *Reproductive Biomedicine Online*. (18)1:43–49.
25. Rajcan-Separovic, E. (2012). Chromosome microarrays in human reproduction. *Human Reproduction Update*. 18(5):555–567.
26. Belkin, Lisa. (2008). "70-year-old woman gives birth." *New York Times*. December 9, 2008.
27. Belkin, Lisa. (2009). "World's oldest mom dies." *New York Times*. July 17, 2009.
28. Paulson, R. (2013). How old is too old to give birth? Available at the USC Fertility website: http://www.uscfertility.org/blog/post/128-how-old-is-too-old-to-give-birth. Accessed January 23, 2013.
29. Bioethics Bytes: Multimedia Resources for Teaching Bioethics. (2009). How old is too old to give birth? Available at: http://bioethicsbytes.wordpress.com/2009/07/27/how-old-is-too-old-to-give-birth/. Accessed January 23, 2013.
30. Ethics Committee of the American Society for Reproductive Medicine. (2005). Fertility preservation and reproduction in cancer patients. *Fertility and Sterility*. 83(6):1622–1628.
31. Ethics Committee of the American Society for Reproductive Medicine. (2013). Mature oocyte cryopreservation: a guideline. *Fertility and Sterility*. 99(1):37–43.

32. Ethics Committee of the American Society for Reproductive Medicine. (2004). Posthumous reproduction. *Fertility and Sterility*. 82(1):S260–262.
33. Strong, C., Gingrich J.R., Kutteh, W.H. (2000). Ethics of postmortem sperm retrieval: Ethics of sperm retrieval after death or persistent vegetative state. *Human Reproduction*. 15(4):739–745.
34. The Ethics Committee of the American Society for Reproduction. (2000). Human somatic cell nuclear transfer (cloning). *Fertility and Sterility*. 74(5):873–876.
35. Roan, S. (2008). "What should be done with excess frozen embryos?" *The Seattle Times*. October 12, 2008. Available at: http://seattletimes.com/html/nationworld/2008257408_embryos12.html. Accessed January 30, 2013.
36. The Ethics Committee of the American Society for Reproduction. (2009). Access to fertility treatment by gays, lesbians, and unmarried persons. *Fertility and Sterility*. 92(4):1190–1193.

4

Testing Children for Adult-Onset Disorders

DAWN C. ALLAIN

Amy is grappling with whether she wants to know if she is at risk for developing Alzheimer disease. However, her brother Peter is an information seeker and planner. Peter has already undergone genetic counseling and testing and was found to have a deleterious mutation in the *PSEN1* gene. Given this information, Peter and his wife met with a financial planner and lawyer to develop a legal and financial plan that will protect his family once he develops symptoms of Alzheimer disease. Peter and his wife also want to plan financially and legally for their children, and they believe that knowing whether Peter is at risk for developing Alzheimer is critical to appropriate planning. Thus, Peter and his wife requested that their 5-year-old son and 8-year-old daughter be tested for the *PSEN1* gene mutation identified in Peter.

Introduction

The utilization of genetic testing in clinical care, research, and through direct-to-consumer testing (as already illustrated in other chapters) raises myriad ethical, social, and legal dilemmas. While there are few ethical dilemmas around the use of genetic testing for the diagnosis or confirmation of a genetic condition in childhood, the ethical implications specifically raised by the application of testing minors for adult-onset genetic diseases have generated a well-documented public and professional discourse.

It is important to note that there are several different reasons for why one might pursue genetic testing in minors. Testing can be performed to confirm a diagnosis and provide information that can be utilized for medical management. According to recent calculations, it is estimated that approximately 4 million newborn children in the United States undergo newborn screening for disorders where early treatment may prevent or reduce morbidity and mortality.[1] In these cases, children are screened within 48 hours of birth and the genetic test result will directly benefit the children because they may then be eligible for early medical interventions such as physical, speech, or occupational therapies, surgeries, special diets, or medications. Other examples of diagnostic testing in childhood include utilizing chromosomal microarrays to delineate an underlying cause of learning disabilities and/or multiple congenital anomalies, allowing for more targeted early childhood services; confirmation of a suspected clinical diagnosis such as Marfan syndrome, which requires ongoing cardiac management; diagnosis of Gaucher disease, where affected individuals can benefit from enzyme replacement therapy; and determining whether an at-risk child has inherited his or her mother's multiple endocrine neoplasia 2B gene mutation and requires prophylactic thyroidectomy. In these cases, where medical management in childhood is impacted, few ethical concerns are raised.

It is when genetic test results do not or cannot impact medical management until later in life that ethical concerns become apparent. One example would be testing a minor to determine if he or she is a carrier of an autosomal recessive or X-linked condition diagnosed in a sibling, such as sickle cell disease or Duchene muscular dystrophy. Even more controversial is the use of genetic testing to determine if a minor is at risk for developing a genetic disorder that will present only in adulthood, regardless of whether there are medical interventions available. Examples of this type of testing include testing a child for mutations in the *BRCA1* or *BRCA2* gene, which if inherited would put her at increased risk for developing breast and/or ovarian cancer in adulthood, or testing for a mutation in a gene that leads to the development of an adult-onset neurodegenerative disease such as Huntington disease. Historically, in these cases the general consensus has been that unless medical intervention could benefit the minor, testing should be deferred until he or she reaches adult status. As such, statements and guidelines have been published by numerous professional organizations stating this position.[1–8] In addition, bioethicists and other healthcare professionals have outlined and rationalized this position by presenting myriad ethical principles that are challenged when considering genetic testing of minors for adult-onset conditions.[9–32]

Interestingly, with the onset of new genetic technology the position of deferring testing until the minor has attained adulthood is being considered again within professional genetic organizations. In addition, consumer advocates have also been requesting more consideration of the rights of parents when deciding whether their children should be tested for adult-onset disorders.

Using the Alzheimer disease case scenario, this chapter will outline the historical perspectives regarding genetic testing for adult-onset diseases in minors and the ethical principles that were addressed by the position statements. In addition, the chapter will explore the current stance regarding the screening and diagnosis of children for adult-onset disorders.

Genetic Testing

Genetic tests for many different diseases are performed in several different settings. This has led to the following categorization of tests: newborn screening, diagnostic testing, carrier testing, prenatal testing, assisted reproductive technologies, predictive testing, and susceptibility testing. For the purpose of this chapter, we will focus on the potential use of predictive/susceptibility testing and carrier testing in minors.

Predictive Testing

Presymptomatic and predictive testing allow for the identification of individuals who are at risk for developing a condition at some point in their lives. Purely defined, predictive testing implies that if an individual tests positive for a disease-causing mutation, he or she will eventually develop the disease at some point in his or her life. The era of predictive genetic testing arose in 1986 when the ability to perform linkage analysis for the DNA markers close to the Huntington disease gene (HTT) became feasible.[34,35] Eventually, in 1993, expansion of the CAG repeat in the *HTT* gene was associated with the development of Huntington disease (HD), and molecular testing without linkage analysis could be performed.[35] Until this discovery, the majority of genetic testing being performed clinically was done to confirm a diagnosis based upon an individual's specific clinical features or results from diagnostic imaging. In regard to Huntington disease, individuals who were at risk had no way to determine if they had inherited the disorder until they presented with clinical symptoms. The identification of the underlying molecular cause of the condition allowed at-risk, asymptomatic individuals the opportunity to undergo genetic analysis of the *HHT* gene to determine whether they were at risk for developing HD before symptoms presented.

Susceptibility gene testing is different from predictive testing in that if an individual is identified as having a mutation in a disease-causing gene, it does not necessarily mean the disease will develop. Genetic testing for mutations in the *BRCA1* and *BRCA2* genes, which are responsible for the rare hereditary breast and ovarian cancer syndrome, is an example of susceptibility gene testing. Those women who test positive for a mutation in the *BRCA1* or *BRCA2* genes have an estimated lifetime risk of 60% to 80% for developing breast cancer and up to a 40% chance of developing ovarian cancer.[36–38] Testing positive for disease-causing mutations confers a *chance* or *likelihood* of developing the disease; however, there are women who test positive for mutations in these genes and never develop breast or ovarian cancer. Unlike Huntington disease, where there is no efficacious treatment or prevention available to those at risk, identification of a cancer susceptibility mutation allows for early cancer screening or preventative surgeries as treatment modalities.

When testing for mutations that cause Huntington disease became available, the ability to test for a condition that had not yet led to clinical symptoms was novel to the genetics profession. This led to the development of very strict protocols for how the provision of genetic counseling, psychological assessment, molecular testing, result disclosure, and follow-up should be carried out.[39,40] The overriding tenet at play in these protocols was respect for autonomy in the individual's decision to test or not. As the identification of other presymptomatic or predictive gene testing became available, the delivery of genetic counseling and testing service often modeled the Huntington disease protocols. Given that concern about the potential impact on an unaffected adult led to the development of strict protocols for the provision of genetic services, it is not surprising that caution when approaching testing in minors was also a prevalent concern. In fact, very early on, questions were raised as to whether an individual who had not yet attained a recognized age of adulthood should be tested for an adult-onset disorder, particularly if there were no medical interventions that could prevent or slow the onset of the condition that would occur later in life. Thus, embedded within the early Huntington disease testing protocols and guidelines was always the statement that HD molecular testing should only be available to an individual who had reached the age of majority. Genetic counseling and testing services in other adult-onset disorders were often modeled on the Huntington disease protocols and, as such, testing of minors for these disorders remained a concern.

Thus, even families with a susceptibility gene mutation that predisposed at-risk individuals to cancer were and still are counseled not to test a minor unless treatment interventions were going to be offered, available, and effective at the time the testing is performed.

Carrier Testing

Molecular testing to identify individuals who carry mutations in genes for autosomal recessive conditions, such as Tay Sachs disease, cystic fibrosis, sickle cell disease, Duchene muscular dystrophy, and other conditions, has been available for over 20 years. Traditionally, carrier testing/screening is performed in adulthood either before conception or early in a pregnancy to enable at-risk couples to make informed reproductive decisions. For example, if someone is a known carrier for cystic fibrosis he or she can have his or her partner undergo carrier testing to determine the likelihood that the couple would have a child affected with cystic fibrosis. If both are found to be carriers of the disorder, then decisions about the use of preimplantation diagnosis, prenatal testing, assisted technologies, pregnancy prevention, or adoption can be considered. Ideally testing is done prior to conceiving a pregnancy, and because of this there are some individuals who suggest that childhood or adolescence may be an appropriate time for carrier testing.

Arguments Against Genetic Testing in Minors

Nonmaleficence

There is a vast body of literature delineating arguments for and against genetic testing in minors. The primary argument against testing a minor for an adult-onset condition is to avoid psychological harm of the minor, which can be equated to the ethical principle of nonmaleficence.[25,27–29,31,41] Studies suggest that deleterious (harmful) genetic results could lead to minors having poor body image, feelings of unworthiness and/or shame, and poor self-esteem.[2,18,19,24,41–46] Well-documented research shows that when adults are informed of their carrier statuses for autosomal recessive conditions they view their health less favorably than those people who are found to be noncarriers.[47,48] Thus, there is concern that minors may be more psychologically vulnerable than adults and, as such, knowledge about carrier or at-risk status may cause harm.[1] Studies have also documented concerns about potential increases in day-to-day or situational anxiety and/or depression.[31,49]

Other potential psychological sequelae include fear of relationship changes, particularly in regard to societal stigmatization and the impact on familial relationships.[24,29,31,41,44,46,49–51] Many researchers and ethicists cite the impact on the parent–child bond as being at risk.[18,31,52] The underlying premise is that if a parent knows that his or her child is at risk for a genetic disease, how the parent treats the child and his or her expectations/hopes for the child's future will change. The concern is that parents will potentially change how they support their children, specifically by withdrawing or limiting resources—emotionally, financially, and physically—from a child who is at risk for developing a disease.[31,46,53] In one review of the literature it was found that some ethicists and researchers believed that parents may remove themselves emotionally from the relationship with their children in order to protect themselves from the knowledge that their children will one day be affected by a genetic disorder or may die from the disease.[54] The relationship between siblings and other family members may also be disrupted when one sibling tests positive and another is negative. Given the literature surrounding the concept of "survivor guilt," it can also be implied that among siblings who have not tested positive there may be feelings of survivor guilt.[30,55,56] In addition, it is possible that feelings of jealousy among siblings may occur if parental–child bonds are disrupted and/or unequally balanced.

While all of these concerns may be justified, there is no evidence-based literature that actually supports the premise that genetic testing for adult-onset disorders in children in fact leads to psychological harm.[54] The lack of evidence is necessarily related to the fact that this type of testing is not being performed in minors or, if it is, it is done rarely. As such, the ability to collect data about outcomes is limited by the low numbers of individuals actually tested. Thus the argument that genetic testing can cause harm, which in turn evokes the ethical principle of nonmaleficence, is really at this time a theoretical concept.

Autonomy

One of the strongest arguments against predictive/carrier testing in a minor evokes the ethical principle of autonomy. The crux of this debate revolves around two major themes tied to an individual's autonomy: testing minors disregards their *future decision-making capacity,* and disclosing results to parents breaches the minor's *confidentiality.*

Future Decision-Making Capacity

The basic premise here is the belief that children and adolescents are not yet capable or mature enough to weigh risks and benefits of decisions regarding genetic testing, nor can they appreciate the long-term impact of their decisions. By delaying genetic testing one is therefore respecting the individual's rights as a future adult (or mature individual) capable of making his or her own informed choices. In the decision *not* to test the nonautonomous minor, one is allowing him or her to be able to determine, at some point in the future, whether he or she wants to be tested and how to utilize this information. At this future point, individuals would have the opportunity to explore the risks, benefits, and limitations of the genetic test and come to a decision about whether they want to pursue genetic testing based upon their current values and beliefs. Hence, the very definition of autonomy is achieved. Testing children for adult-onset disorders or carrier status undermines or limits future autonomous decision-making capacity.

Confidentiality

While perhaps not obviously related, confidentiality is often raised as an underpinning in the ethical principle of autonomy. Testing a minor for a genetic disorder violates his or her confidentiality because the test result will be shared with the parents without the child's consent. The child also has no control over with whom the parents share the genetic test results. Disclosure of these results by a healthcare provider to the parents, or by the parents with other individuals, without express consent of the minor violates the minor's autonomous right to privacy.[53] The disclosure of these results could lead to both familial and social stigmatization, as well as other psychological sequelae cited earlier. Tied into the concern with confidentiality is the fear of genetic discrimination.[50] Testing the minor and documenting the at-risk status of the individual in medical records carries a risk of disclosure of this information to third parties, which could put the minor at risk for future insurance or employment discrimination.

Beneficence

While the tenet of "doing no harm" is a primary argument for the avoidance of predictive and presymptomatic testing in minors, another argument against carrier testing or predictive testing in minors is that there would be no immediate medical benefit for the minor.[41,51,57–59] For example, if a minor undergoes genetic testing for Alzheimer disease there are currently no medical interventions that would be utilized in childhood which would prevent or reduce the likelihood that the minor will develop this condition at any point in life. In the case of hereditary breast and ovarian cancer syndrome, even if a minor tested positive for a mutation in one of the *BRCA* genes, mammography is still not recommended until she reaches the age of 25 years. In this argument, by not testing a minor one is actually helping the minor *avoid* all of the potential harms delineated previously in this chapter such as the potential risk of breach of confidentiality, denying the minor the right to future decision making, and psychosocial harms. Thus, the principle of beneficence must be considered in the argument against testing minors. In addition, it is one of the primary motivations in a variety of professional position statements about testing in minors.

Professional Position Statements and Guidelines

Given the concerns highlighted above, many professional organizations have published position statements regarding genetic testing in minors. The earliest of these was published by the United Kingdom Clinical Genetics Society (CGS) in 1994, shortly after the Huntington disease gene was discovered, and delineates six conclusions and/or recommendations regarding genetic testing in children.[2] The principle message was that predictive genetic testing of minors is necessary and appropriate when the onset of a condition occurs in childhood or when there are implications for medical management. However, if the testing does not lead to changes in medical management or interventions, then the position statement advises that predictive testing in minors should be avoided. Several professional societies subsequently developed "points to consider" documents or position statements regarding the ethical, legal, and psychosocial implications of genetic testing in children and adolescents.[5–8,28,60] The majority of these draw conclusions similar to those of the CGS, stating that the primary motivation for genetic testing in minors should be timely medical benefit, and if the medical benefit is unclear or if interventions will not occur until the minor attains adulthood then the justification for testing is not as persuasive. Of interest is the American College of Medical Genetics and Genomics (ACMG) recent publication recommending that when whole-exome or whole-genome sequencing* is performed, the clinical laboratories performing these tests should report mutations in 57 specific genes.[33] The genes selected by ACMG include highly penetrant disorders for which treatment/prevention exists. However, if this testing is done in a minor, disclosure of these results contradicts ACMG's own joint recommendation with the American Pediatric Association (APA) regarding avoidance of testing in minors.[28] This statement is particularly concerning in the context of testing minors, given that a large number of the diseases caused by these genes are of adult onset.

Arguments for Genetic Testing in Minors

While there are many professional guidelines and statements regarding limiting or deferring predictive and carrier testing in minors, there is also a vast literature documenting reasons in favor of such testing raised in the context of ethical principles.

Autonomy

One argument addresses the concept of parental rights, which is based on the premise that parents have the authority to make medical decisions on behalf of their children for all other medical treatments and interventions.[24,45,53,61] In this argument, authority is

* Whole genome sequencing (WGS) is a laboratory technique that identifies the entire DNA of an organism and includes analysis of all introns, exons, and mitochondrial DNA. Whole exome sequencing (WES), like WGS, is a laboratory technique. However, WES only targets the coding regions of the genome. Both techniques are used in an attempt to identify disease-causing genetic variants.

given to parents because it is believed that minors do not have the cognitive ability or maturity to make complicated decisions, medically related or otherwise. This presumes lack of autonomy in the child. As such, it can conversely be viewed as *parental autonomy*, as parents have reached the legal age of majority (or are legally emancipated as in the case of minors who have given birth). It is also important to note that there is case law in the United States that has reinforced parental rights to make decisions for their children and family. It has been argued that these court rulings can be used to justify parental decision making about genetic testing for their children.[45,53] The argument of parental autonomy as a reason for pursuing genetic testing in minors is also based upon the tenet that parents will act in the best interests of their children.[19,25,61,62] In fact, one commentary published in 2007 emphatically states that parents who want to pursue genetic testing are doing so to make realistic future plans regarding treatment, management, and psychological support for their children.[43] In addition, several studies have shown that following newborn screening, parents want carrier status to be reported to them and that they plan to discuss their child's carrier status with the child at some point in the future, given that it has implications for the minor's future reproductive risks.[63,64] One could also argue that having lived with the genetic disorder themselves or within the family, parents are most likely capable of coping with the psychological and medical implications of the disorder and thereby are the best resources for their at-risk child.

Proponents of testing in minors also make the argument that there are young children and adolescents who are capable of making their own informed decisions.[54,62,65,66] Therefore, delaying the option of genetic testing for adult-onset disorders or carrier status is actually denying or limiting their ability to make autonomous decisions.[62,67] Others have argued that not testing minors also limits their current autonomy and development because if they are untested they will not have the necessary knowledge to adapt and integrate their disease status.[44] It is important to note that none of the authors who cite that minors have the cognitive ability to make their own decisions refute the concerns cited for delaying testing. Their argument of support for testing is based wholly on the concept that a minor, when appropriately counseled and provided with resources, can make an informed choice and maintain autonomous decision making. If children have confirmation of their at-risk status, then they may be more likely to be empowered and take an active role in maintaining their health. This may increase the likelihood that the adolescent or minor would ultimately adhere to treatment and management guidelines, since he or she was responsible for the testing decision. Elger et al. go as far as to suggest that respecting adolescents' autonomous decision making regarding genetic testing could lead to an increase in their overall self-esteem and accentuate their coping strategies.[65] One could also argue that allowing minors to make autonomous decisions minimizes or avoids the potential of healthcare provider paternalism in the decision-making process. Interestingly, the current NSGC position statement on genetic testing of minors for adult-onset conditions actually supports the concept of the minor's autonomy.[68] While it recommends deferral of predictive genetic testing of minors for adult-onset genetic disease whenever possible to when the minor attains adulthood, it also allows for the individual to make his or her own decision about testing based upon personally developed beliefs, values, preferences, and situation. This implies that should a minor or parent of a minor seek testing for an adult-onset condition, it is conceivable that the testing could occur provided he or she has carefully weighed the benefits, limitations, and risks for that particular situation and with the appropriate stakeholders involved.

Beneficence

Since one of the primary arguments against predictive/presymptomatic or carrier genetic testing in minors is related to the ethical principle of nonmaleficence in regards to psychological harm, it is not hard to understand why the principle of beneficence would be tied to the psychological benefits of testing. Using the arguments delineated above for not testing, one can make the same arguments for testing a minor. For example, those supporting genetic testing in a minor would suggest knowledge of at-risk status can positively affect body image and self- esteem.[12,43,45,54] There is also literature that suggests undergoing genetic testing may decrease a minor's anxiety and risk for depression.[19,31,54] For example, the individual is now aware of what his or her actual risk is instead of having a perception of risk. This can allow the minor to develop and incorporate coping strategies to deal with the risk status (whether receiving a negative or positive genetic test result). Knowledge of test results can alleviate or diminish the level of uncertainty for the minor and perhaps reduce overall anxiety. In addition to the psychological benefit to the minor, there is literature to support that testing in a minor may also provide benefits to the parents. Testing could help decrease anxiety for the parents, again with the idea of known risk versus the uncertainty of perceived risk.[69] Testing also allows time for both the minor and the parent to adjust psychologically and emotionally to the implication of the test results. It may also allow for more realistic parental expectations and have a positive effect on family dynamics.[43,54] Proponents for testing a minor also argue that individuals who test positive may benefit from early lifestyle modifications. For example, someone at risk for cancer may elect not to smoke tobacco products, may be more diligent about exercise, and may follow a different diet. Knowing results allows for future life planning, including deliberative career choices, long-term disability planning, and establishing financial resources.

Application to Case Study

Mutations in *PSEN1* are associated with complete penetrance by age 65 years, with the majority of individuals diagnosed before

60 years of age. Given this clinical presentation, testing for *PSEN1* gene mutations in asymptomatic individuals is considered predictive/presymptomatic testing. However, testing positive for a disease-causing mutation does not predict age of onset, severity of the symptoms, or progression of the disease. Additionally, as treatment for Alzheimer disease is currently supportive and symptom-managed, there are currently no early interventions or therapies available for unaffected at-risk individuals.

In the case study presented at the beginning of the chapter, Peter is described as an information seeker and planner. He has already sought genetic counseling and testing and is known to carry a deleterious mutation in the *PSEN1* gene. Now Peter and his wife are requesting genetic testing in their two children, ages 5 and 8. Applying the information presented in this chapter, the primary argument *for* testing Peter's children would be to provide the family with psychological relief, as not knowing their at-risk status may be providing undue psychological anxiety for Peter and his wife. If the children test negative it reduces the likelihood of them developing Alzheimer disease to the general population risk, and that knowledge could provide reassurance for the family. In addition, knowledge about whether the children are at risk could allow for long-term financial and estate planning for the family, ensuring that the parents and children are taken care of in the future. Of course there is also the argument that this knowledge may positively impact Peter and his wife's relationship with the children, particularly if the children are found not to be at risk.

Alternatively, the primary argument for *not* testing Peter's children is that it removes the autonomy of the children to choose whether they actually want to know their at-risk status. Given that there is no medical intervention available at all for the condition, one could argue that there is no benefit to testing the children at this time. In addition, although not explored in detail in this chapter, test results could lead to interfamilial and intrafamilial social stigmatization, employment discrimination, and insurance discrimination.

Healthcare professionals would need to communicate to Peter and his wife in a clear, concise manner the various risks associated with testing weighed against the benefits of testing. Utilizing professional guidelines and position statements, one could argue that in this setting, testing the minor might actually do harm because of the lack of possibility for medical intervention, risk for discrimination, and potential psychological harms. One would hope that with appropriate counseling and discussion the family could come to a decision that would be accepted by all.

REFERENCES

1. Committee on Bioethics, Committee on Genetics, and the ACMG Social and Ethical Legal Issues Committee. (2013). Ethical and policy issues in genetic testing and screening of children. *Pediatrics*. 131(3):620–622.
2. Clarke, A. Working Party of the Clinical Genetics Society (UK). (1994). The genetic testing of children. *Journal of Medical Genetics*. 31(10):785–797.
3. International Huntington Association and the World Federation of Neurology Research Group on Huntington's Chorea. (1994). Guidelines for the molecular genetics predictive test in Huntington's disease. *Journal of Medical Genetics*. 31(7):555–559.
4. European Society of Human Genetics. (2009). Genetic testing in asymptomatic minors: Recommendations of the European Society of Human Genetics. *European Journal of Human Genetics*. 17(6):720–721.
5. American Society of Human Genetics Board of Directors, American College of Medical Genetics and Genomics Board of Directors. (1995). Points to consider: ethical, legal, and psychosocial implications of genetic testing in children and adolescents. *American Journal of Human Genetics* 57(5):1233–1241.
6. Arbour, L., Committee CPSB. (2003). Guidelines for genetic testing of healthy children. A joint statement with the Candadian College of Medical Geneticists. *Paediatrics & Child Health* 8(1):42–45.
7. Bioethics Committee. (2001). Ethical issues with genetic testing in pediatrics. *Pediatrics* 107(6):1451–1455.

8. Borry, P., Evers-Kiebooms, G., Cornel, M.C., Clarke, A., Dierickx, K. (2009). Genetic testing in asymptomatic minors: background considerations towards ESHG Recommendations. *European Journal of Human Genetics.* 17(6):711–719.
9. Borry, P., Nys, H., Dierickx, K. (2007). Carrier testing in minors: conflicting views. *Nature Reviews Genetics.* 8(11):828.
10. Campbell, E., Ross, L.F. (2003). Professional and personal attitudes about access and confidentiality in the genetic testing of children: a pilot study. *Genetic Testing.* 7(2):123–130.
11. Clancy, T. (2010). A clinical perspective on ethical arguments around prenatal diagnosis and preimplantation genetic diagnosis for later onset inherited cancer predispositions. *Familial Cancer.* 9(1):9–14.
12. Elger, B.S., Harding, T.W. (2000). Testing adolescents for a hereditary breast cancer gene (BRCA1): respecting their autonomy is in their best interest. *Archives of Pediatrics & Adolescent Medicine.* 154(2):113–119.
13. Fresneau, B., Brugières, L., Caron, O., Moutel, G. (2013). Ethical issues in presymptomatic genetic testing for minors: A dilemma in Li-Fraumeni syndrome. *Journal of Genetic Counseling.* 22(3):315–322.
14. Hanson, J.W., Thomson, E.J. (2000). Genetic testing in children: ethical and social points to consider. *Pediatric Annals.* 29(5):285–291.
15. Harper, P.S., Clarke, A. (1990). Should we test children for "adult" genetic diseases? *Lancet.* 335(8699):1205–1206.
16. Huggins, M., Bloch, M., Kanani, S., Quarrell, O.W., Theilman, J., Hedrick. A, et al. (1990). Ethical and legal dilemmas arising during predictive testing for adult-onset disease: the experience of Huntington disease. *American Journal of Human Genetics.* 47(1):4–12.
17. Lebel, R.R. (1995). Genetic testing for children and adolescents. *Journal of the American Medical Association.* 273(14):1089; author reply 90.
18. Lessick, M., Faux, S. (1998). Implications of genetic testing of children and adolescents. *Holistic Nursing Practice.* 12(3):38–46.
19. Mand, C., Gillam, L., Delatycki, M.B., Duncan, R.E. (2012). Predictive genetic testing in minors for late-onset conditions: a

chronological and analytical review of the ethical arguments. *Journal of Medical Ethics.* 38(9):519–524.
20. Marteau, T.M. (1994). The genetic testing of children. *Journal of Medical Genetics.* 31(10):743.
21. Martinez, W. (1998). Genetic testing of children and adolescents: ethical, legal and psychosocial implications. *Princeton Journal of Bioethics.* 1(1):65–75.
22. Otlowski M. An exploration of the legal and socio-ethical implications of predictive genetic testing of children (2004) *Australian Journal of Family Law* 18(2): 147–169.
23. Patenaude, A.F. (1996). The genetic testing of children for cancer susceptibility: ethical, legal, and social issues. *Behavioral Sciences & the Law.* 14(4):393–410.
24. Rhodes, R. (2006). Why test children for adult-onset genetic diseases? *The Mount Sinai Journal of Medicine.* 73(3):609–616.
25. Robertson, S., Savulescu, J. (2001). Is there a case in favour of predictive genetic testing in young children? *Bioethics.* 15(1):26–49.
26. Robertson, S.P., Kerruish, N. (2012). Resolving the impasse on predictive genetic testing in minors: will more evidence be the solution? *Journal of Medical Ethics.* 38(9):525–526.
27. Ross, L.F. (2004). Should children and adolescents undergo genetic testing? *Pediatric Annals.* 33(11):762–769.
28. Ross, L.F., Saal, H.M., David, K.L., Anderson, R.R., American Academy of Pediatrics, American College of Medical Genetics and Genomics. (2013). Technical report: ethical and policy issues in genetic testing and screening of children. *Genetics in Medicine.* 15(3):234–245.
29. Savulescu, J. (2001). Predictive genetic testing in children. *The Medical Journal of Australia.* 175(7):379–381.
30. Uzych, L. (1995). Genetic testing for children and adolescents. *Journal of the American Medical Association.* 273(14):1089–1090.
31. Wertz, D.C., Fanos, J.H., Reilly, P.R. (1994). Genetic testing for children and adolescents. Who decides? *Journal of the American Medical Association.* 272(11):875–881.
32. Sharpe, N.F. (1993). Presymptomatic testing for Huntington disease: is there a duty to test those under the age of eighteen years? *American Journal of Medical Genetics.* 46(2):250–253.
33. Green, R.C., Berg, J.S., Grody, W.W., Kalia, S.S., Korf, B.R., Martin, C.L., et al. (2013). ACMG recommendations for reporting

of incidental findings in clinical exome and genome sequencing. *Genetics in Medicine.* 15(7):565–574.

34. Gusella, J.F., Wexler, N.S., Conneally, P.M., Naylor, S.L., Anderson, M.A., Tanzi, R.E., et al. (1983). A polymorphic DNA marker genetically linked to Huntington's disease. *Nature.* 306(5940):234–238.
35. MacDonald, M.E., Ambrose, C.M., Duyao, M.P., Myers, R.H., Lin, C., Srinidhi, L., et al. (1993). A novel gene containing a trinucleotide repeat that is expanded and unstable on Huntington's disease chromosomes. *Cell* 72(6):971–983.
36. Antoniou, A., Pharoah, P.D., Narod, S., Risch, H.A., Eyfjord, J.E., Hopper, J.L., et al. (2003). Average risks of breast and ovarian cancer associated with BRCA1 or BRCA2 mutations detected in case series unselected for family history: a combined analysis of 22 studies. *American Journal of Human Genetics.* 72(5):1117–11130.
37. Ford, D., Easton, D.F., Bishop, D.T., Narod, S.A., Goldgar, D.E. Breast Cancer Linkage Consortium. (1994). Risks of cancer in BRCA1-mutation carriers. *Lancet.* 343(8899):692–695.
38. King, M.C., Marks, J.H., Mandell, J.B. (2003). Breast and ovarian cancer risks due to inherited mutations in BRCA1 and BRCA2. *Science.* 302(5645):643–646.
39. World Federation of Neurology: Research Committee. Research Group on Huntington's chorea. (1989). Ethical issues policy statement on Huntington's disease molecular genetics predictive test. *Journal of the Neurological Sciences.* 94(1–3):327–332.
40. Went, L. (1990). Ethical issues policy statement on Huntington's disease molecular genetics predictive test. *Journal of Medical Genetics.* 27:34–38.
41. Bloch, M., Hayden, M.R. (1990). Opinion: predictive testing for Huntington disease in childhood: challenges and implications. *American Journal of Human Genetics.* 46(1):1–4.
42. Lucassen, A.M., Houlston, R.S. (2000). Clinical geneticists' attitudes and practice towards testing for breast cancer susceptibility genes. *Journal of Medical Genetics.* 37(2):157–160.
43. Malpas, P.J. (2008). Predictive genetic testing of children for adult-onset diseases and psychological harm. *Journal of Medical Ethics.* 34(4):275–278.
44. Duncan, R.E. (2004). Predictive genetic testing in young people: When is it appropriate? *Journal of Paediatrics and Child Health.* 40(11):593–595.

45. Pelias, M.K. (2006). Genetic testing of children for adult-onset diseases: is testing in the child's best interests? *The Mount Sinai Journal of Medicine.* 73(3):605–608.
46. Ross, L.F., Moon, M.R. (2000). Ethical issues in genetic testing of children. *Archives of Pediatrics & Adolescent Medicine.* 154(9):873–879.
47. Rowley, P.T. (1989). Parental receptivity to neonatal sickle trait identification. *Pediatrics.* 83(5 Pt 2):891–893.
48. Marteau, T.M., van Duijn, M., Ellis, I. (1992). Effects of genetic screening on perceptions of health: a pilot study. *Journal of Medical Genetics.* 29(1):24–26.
49. Cappelli, M., Verma, S., Korneluk, Y., Hunter, A., Tomiak, E., Allanson, J, et al. (2005). Psychological and genetic counseling implications for adolescent daughters of mothers with breast cancer. *Clinical Genetics.* 67(6):481–491.
50. Harel, A., Abuelo, D., Kazura, A. (2003). Adolescents and genetic testing: what do they think about it? *The Journal of Adolescent Health.* 33(6):489–494.
51. Welkenhuysen, M., Evers-Kiebooms, G. (2003). Predictive genetic testing for breast cancer and Huntington's disease: the opinions of midwives and nurses in Flanders. *Community Genetics.* 6(2):104–113.
52. Duncan, R.E., Savulescu, J., Gillam, L., Williamson, R., Delatycki, M.B. (2005). An international survey of predictive genetic testing in children for adult onset conditions. *Genetics in Medicine.* 7(6):390–396.
53. Holland, J. (1997). Should parents be permitted to authorize genetic testing for their children? *Family Law Quarterly.* 31(2):321–353.
54. Duncan, R.E., Delatycki, M.B. (2006). Predictive genetic testing in young people for adult-onset conditions: where is the empirical evidence? *Clinical Genetics.* 69(1):8–16; discussion 7–20.
55. Cummings, S. (2000). The genetic testing process: how much counseling is needed? *Journal of Clinical Oncology.* 18(21 Suppl):60S–4S.
56. Lerman, C., Daly, M., Masny, A., Balshem, A. (1994). Attitudes about genetic testing for breast-ovarian cancer susceptibility. *Journal of Clinical Oncology.* 12(4):843–850.
57. Welkenhuysen, M., Evers-Kiebooms, G. (2003). The reactions of general practitioners, nurses and midwives in Flanders concerning

breast cancer risks in a high-risk situation. *Community Genetics.* 6(4):206–213.

58. Borry, P., Fryns, J.P., Schotsmans, P., Dierickx, K. (2006). Carrier testing in minors: a systematic review of guidelines and position papers. *European Journal of Human Genetics.* 14(2):133–138.
59. Borry, P., Goffin, T., Nys, H., Dierickx, K. (2008). Attitudes regarding predictive genetic testing in minors: A survey of European clinical geneticists. *American Journal of Medical Genetics.* Part C: Seminars in Medical Genetics 148C(1):78–83.
60. National Society of Genetic Counselors' resolutions ballot: prenatal and childhood testing for adult-onset disorders. Position Statement. Wallingford, PA; 1995.
61. Borry, P., Goffin, T., Nys, H., Dierickx, K. (2008). Predictive genetic testing in minors for adult-onset genetic diseases. *Mount Sinai Journal of Medicine.* 75(3):287–296.
62. Clayton, E.W. (1997). Genetic testing in children. *The Journal of Medicine and Philosophy.* 22(3):233–251.
63. Oliver, S., Dezateux, C., Kavanagh, J., Lempert, T., Stewart, R. (2004). Disclosing to parents newborn carrier status identified by routine blood spot screening. *The Cochrane Database of Systematic Reviews.* October 18(4):CD003859.
64. Laird, L., Dezateux, C., Anionwu, E.N. (1996). Fortnightly Review: Neonatal screening for sickle cell disorders: what about the carrier infants? *British Medical Journal.* 313(7054):407–411.
65. Elger, B.S., Harding, T.W. (2000). Pediatric forum: genetic testing of adolescents: is it in their best interest? *Archives of Pediatrics & Adolescent Medicine.* 154(8): 850–852.
66. Cohen, C.B. (1998). Wrestling with the future: should we test children for adult-onset genetic conditions? *Kennedy Institute of Ethics Journal.* 8(2):111–130.
67. Malpas, P.J. (2006). Why tell asymptomatic children of the risk of an adult-onset disease in the family but not test them for it? *Journal of Medical Ethics.* 32(11):639–42.
68. National Society of Genetic Counselors. (2012). Genetic testing of minors for adult-onset conditions. Available at: http://nsgc.org/p/bl/et/blogid=47&blogaid=28
69. Fryer, A. (1995). Genetic testing of children. *Archives of Disease in Childhood.* 73(2):97–99.

5

These Are Not the Genes You Are Looking For

Incidental Findings Identified as a Result of Genetic Testing

CURTIS R. COUGHLIN II

Incidental findings can occur in any medical discipline. Until recently, incidental findings identified as a result of genetic testing were relatively rare. The field of medical genetics has recently undergone a paradigm shift. Both the genetic researcher and clinician have adopted the use of untargeted genetic analysis such as exome sequencing, and a "genome first" approach to disease identification has started to emerge. The unbiased nature of genomic testing has identified new genetic syndromes and redefined previous genotype–phenotype relationships, but the frequency of incidental findings has dramatically increased as a result. A recent *Science* article stated that the debate surrounding return of these incidental findings "... is arguably the most pressing issue in genetics today."[1]

In this chapter the term *incidental finding* will refer to any genetic result that is not related to the primary reason for genetic testing. This is the broadest possible definition, as many current definitions of incidental findings also emphasize the medical or social implication of the result. Incidental findings include results that have a high clinical significance (e.g., cancer predisposition syndrome), findings of questionable medical and legal significance (e.g., consanguinity), and findings with reproductive implications (e.g., misattributed paternity). In order to identify an incidental finding, one must also be able to recognize the primary indication for testing. This may not be difficult in a targeted research study (e.g., subjects with intractable epilepsy) or clinical testing (e.g., a patient with multiple congenital anomalies) and may be impossible if genomic testing is pursued in a healthy individual. In this chapter we will emphasize results that are incidental to a primary reason for testing, although the reader could extrapolate the general information in this chapter to results identified in a healthy individual.

The terms *incidental finding*[2] and *incidentaloma*[3] have been used for over four decades, although there has been increasing criticism that the descriptor "incidental" minimalizes the significance of a genetic result that may have life-altering implications. Many alternative terms have been suggested, such as non-incidental secondary findings, secondary variants, unanticipated results, unexpected results, and unsought-for findings.[4,5] Terminology is not as important as ensuring that all stakeholders understand the expectations once an incidental finding is identified. Each suggested term has its own shortcoming, and the rather wide acceptance of the term *incidental finding* perpetuates it as the de facto descriptor (including in this chapter).

The ethical dilemma surrounding the return of incidental findings may not be immediately obvious to the reader. After all, respect for persons (autonomy) is a central tenet of genetic counseling, which is evidenced by the emphasis on genetic education for patients and informed consent. As a result, there is a natural tendency toward disclosure of results. In general, recommendations to disclose incidental findings are strongest when there is known clinical utility of the finding, and caution is recommended when a genetic finding has unclear significance or when the subject is a minor.[6] Not everyone is in favor of "full disclosure" of incidental findings, with concerns that reporting all results to all individuals could provoke anxiety or result in possible genetic stigmatization. This has led many to suggest specific types of results that should be returned[7] and others to list those disorders where a higher moral obligation to return results exists.[8,9]

Although such recommendations are helpful, often the decision to disclose an incidental finding has significant contextual nuances and does not fit into a predefined category. Genetic providers are quite familiar with results that have ambiguous medical implications and are skilled at navigating such difficult social situations. The reader should use the information in this chapter, and the reference material within, to understand the ethical concerns surrounding incidental findings identified through genetic testing. This chapter should serve as a guide and should emphasize general principles surrounding the decision to return an incidental finding, as opposed to a list of what constitutes a medically significant and therefore returnable result.

Ethical Concepts

Many of the ethical issues that arise as a result of untargeted genetic testing are fundamental to the field of genetics. Ethical concerns surrounding misattributed paternity and presymptomatic testing of minors are the cornerstones of ethical discussions held in every genetics training program. Examining incidental findings through ethical concepts that are familiar, such as principlism, will aid the reader when faced with the dilemma of whether to disclose an incidental finding. The concept of principlism provides a pragmatic approach to those ethical dilemmas that the clinician may face. Principlism states that four cardinal principles (autonomy, nonmaleficence, beneficence and justice) can guide the clinician in identifying salient features of a case and the appropriate response.[10] Although many have noted that principlism alone is often unhelpful to the trainee,[11] as well as being fairly narrow and constricted for complex ethical dilemmas,[12] the concept of principlism still dominates current bioethics training in most medical and graduate programs.

Beneficence

The strongest argument in favor of disclosure of incidental findings involves those results that have a well-defined risk to the individual and may be treatable or preventable.[13,14] The ethical concept of beneficence supports the recommendation to disclose a medically actionable result to a patient, and current guidelines have rather uniformly supported the recommendation to return incidental findings that are clinically significant and medically actionable.

The patient's best interest is a very important concept in clinical care but not always assumed in research. Although there is always care to reduce possible harm to a research subject, the primary aim of research is generalizable knowledge and not patient care. Researchers may have had limited clinical contact with research subjects and may have had minimal experience counseling patients about results. Both clinicians and researchers may have limited experience with an incidental finding that is outside their areas of expertise. Although there are significant differences between clinical and research testing that should not be understated, the return of medically actionable incidental findings is recommended regardless of clinical or research testing. In fact, as early as 1999 the National Bioethics Advisory Commission (NBAC) recommended that *research* results be disclosed to subjects if the results were scientifically valid, had significant health implications, and a course of action to treat such concerns was available (http://bioethics.georgetown.edu/nbac/hbm.pdf).

Most of the current recommendations concerning the return of incidental findings have focused on those results that are clinically significant and medically actionable and therefore benefit the patient when disclosed. It is possible to extend the concept of beneficence beyond results that are deemed medically actionable. Patients may value results that have reproductive implications as much as results that have future health implications. After all, a primary aim of medical genetics is "…enabling people and families with a genetic disadvantage to live and reproduce as normally as possible."[15] It is important to evaluate what is the primary aim of the genetic test. If the aim is to provide a patient an accurate recurrence risk for reproductive decision making, then findings that alter recurrence risk may not be incidental at all. It is also not difficult to imagine that the primary aim of a genetic test may be defined differently by the clinician (or researcher) and the patient (or subject).

Although many incidental findings may provide a significant benefit to patients, not all incidental findings can be classified as providing a benefit.[16] Indeed, results that may have important reproductive implications in one situation could have devastating social effects in another situation such as the identification of misattributed paternity (Box 5.1). And those findings that have the potential for harm should require further evaluation. The balancing between benefits (beneficence) and risks of genetic testing (nonmaleficence), described below, will continue to play a role in whether untargeted genetic testing is pursued and whether to disclose incidental findings that are ascertained as a result.

Nonmaleficence

The majority of incidental findings will not have well-defined medical risk and will therefore have limited immediate benefit for the patient. As a result, many caution against the disclosure of incidental findings due to the potential harm that may result. Such harm could result when there is limited understanding of the data, limited access to a "genomic expert" to disclose a result, and the possibility of disclosing a disruptive or undesired result.[17,18] Concern about possibly causing harm, and therefore advocating for nondisclosure, emphasizes the ethical concept of nonmaleficence or "do no harm."

In the majority of incidental findings there will be incomplete understanding of the result and the risk to patient. In this way genomic incidental findings continue to be similar to those incidental findings identified through neuroimaging, where there is a relatively low rate of incidental findings that have had clinical significance. The limited medical benefit and the presumptive increased anxiety of knowing that "something" was identified has led many to favor nondisclosure of results with limited clinical utility. In order to lower possible anxiety for the patient, disclosure of the incidental finding would require discussion with an expert qualified to interpret that result. Not all genetic testing requires a trained genetics provider, since many cardiologists, neurologists, oncologists, and so on are genetics experts within their specific field of study. Yet in general there are relatively few experts with whom to discuss these findings and, in some geographic areas, access is significantly limited. By definition an incidental finding is outside the primary indication for testing or the research aim and therefore possibly outside the expertise of the ordering healthcare provider.

Incidental findings may also be disruptive to a patient's genetic identity or his/her current situation. By favoring disclosure of all results, a genetic provider would be interfering with the patient's "right not to know." Voluntariness, the hallmark of informed consent in genetic testing, emphasizes the patient's right not to know a result. Following genetic education, the patient elects either to know (accept testing) or not to know (decline testing) a specific result.

Autonomy

Respect for persons is a central tenet of genetic counseling and is embodied by the emphasis on education of patients and informed consent prior to genetic testing. The principle of autonomy emphasizes that patients be completely informed so that they can make the best possible decisions for themselves. Most argue that it is during this pretest education phase that patients will be able to make informed decisions and agree to a specific plan concerning identification and return of incidental findings.[5]

Ideally the provider will have discussed the possibility of an incidental finding with the patient, and the patient will have declared his/her preference about disclosure of the result. With targeted testing this ideal may be possible, as one can anticipate the types of results that might arise and counsel the patient on the impact of such results. With untargeted testing it would be impossible to discuss every potential incidental finding during pretest counseling. It would be possible, however, to discuss the various *types* of incidental findings that may arise and ascertain the patient's general preference. Unfortunately, informed consent and pretest education will not occur in every situation, as genetic testing has become rather ubiquitous among medical disciplines. It is not hard to imagine a situation where a patient is not even aware that untargeted genetic testing was performed, let alone have had an opportunity to declare his/her preferences surrounding disclosure of incidental findings.

Incidental Findings

When clinical genetic testing is performed there is an expectation that a result will be returned to the patient, and there is typically a preexisting relationship between the healthcare provider and the patient. Clinical laboratories follow standards to ensure quality laboratory testing. As a result, clinical testing provides an ideal model for both the identification of and the return of incidental findings. Current recommendations surrounding disclosure of incidental findings also focus on the clinical utility of the result, with further emphasis on clinical testing.

Many have attempted to categorize which incidental findings would meet the definition of "a result with high clinical utility." In 2012, 16 well-respected genetic providers were surveyed about 99 common conditions to determine if there was agreement concerning which incidental findings should be returned to an ordering physician.[8] There was considerable concordance between specialists, with unanimous agreement to return incidental findings in 21/99 conditions identified in adults and 4/99 conditions identified in minors. But despite agreement on a few conditions, in general there was significant discordance about whether to disclose most of the incidental findings. Similarly, the American College of Medical Genetics and Genomics (ACMG) appointed a working group to evaluate those incidental findings where an obligation would exist for disclosure. The ACMG working group specifically evaluated incidental findings that would be identified following *clinical* testing, and recommended disclosure if an incidental finding was found in any of 58 genes representing 27 conditions.[9]

A consensus has started to emerge concerning the obligation to return incidental findings that meet a specific criterion of severity and are medically actionable. This is not a new paradigm for clinical laboratories, as known and clinically actionable genes are the primary reasons healthcare providers order clinical testing. The aims of research testing are often quite divergent from the goal of clinical testing. Many research studies are aimed at a specific hypothesis that would not include analysis of such "actionable" genes. These results could still be incidentally found by researchers, although some argue that researchers have the same obligation to find (i.e., search for) and disclose medically actionable results.[20]

Various agencies such as the NBAC; National Heart, Lung and Blood Institute; and Canadian Tri-Council have stated that researchers have a duty to disclose actionable results to research subjects once identified, although there is limited discussion on the researchers' obligations to search for such findings.[21,22] In a survey of 107 genomic scientists identified through Canadian research associations, 36% of respondents agreed that researchers had a responsibility to examine genomic data for specific incidental findings, and the majority (78%) agreed that incidental findings with potential clinical significance should be returned to a subject.[19]

Although many research studies involve a clinician-scientist, typically research studies are lead by investigators who have a limited clinical relationship with the research subject. Many research samples are de-identified, and until recently the majority of genetic-based research studies included informed consent forms that specifically stated that genetic results would not be returned.[1] The anonymity of research samples is often a significant barrier to returning incidental findings. Research laboratories are not typically accredited by CLIA or other applicable accrediting agencies unless the laboratory also has a clinical component. There would be significant legal implications if research results are incorrect, and most advocate that research results should be validated in a clinical laboratory. Although this is a fairly common recommendation, few have discussed whether disclosure of the result would occur before validation of the finding or after testing is sent to a clinical laboratory.

Various stakeholders are starting to make recommendations concerning disclosure of incidental findings. A consensus is starting to emerge that results that have the potential to benefit a patient and have a low likelihood of causing harm should be disclosed to a patient. Yet the increasing adoption of untargeted genetic testing and the increasing knowledge of genotype–phenotype relationships will only increase the incidental findings that meet this criterion for disclosure. By using currently accepted criteria and examining whole genome data in 36 individuals, one group estimated that over 11,000 variants today and over 16,000 variants by the year 2015 would meet the criteria for disclosure.[23] Just as a new paradigm has emerged in genetic testing, a new method of incorporating genetic counseling will need to materialize (Box 5.2).

BOX 5.1 Case Example: Misattributed Paternity

Although large-scale genetic testing may be rather new, genetic providers are quite familiar with the original genetic incidental finding: misattributed paternity. Misattributed paternity, or false paternity, refers to a situation where a man is incorrectly assumed to be the biological father of a child. Typically this result is identified after primary testing for other indications such as parental studies for an autosomal recessive condition, prenatal testing, and testing prior to organ transplantation from a related donor.[24,25]

Although misattributed paternity is an often-discussed ethical dilemma, it is rarely identified as a result of genetic testing. Historically, healthcare providers are taught a misattributed paternity rate of 10%–15%, although this is often a result of anecdotes or oral traditions.[26] It is difficult to estimate an accurate rate of misattributed paternity due to the delicate nature of the information. For men who are relatively sure that they are biological fathers, it appears that the misattributed paternity rate is significantly lower (1%–3%) than previously thought.[27]

Genetic providers have typically preferred nondisclosure of misattributed paternity, or at least limited disclosure of the finding. The position to withhold or limit disclosure (to only the mother) was supported by a 1994 Institute of Medicine Committee on Assessing Genetic Risks.[28] Others have suggested that what is important to disclose is the information directly related to testing (i.e., recurrence risk for the couple) and not to disclose the incidental finding.[29] In a series of surveys, the vast majority of medical geneticists, clinical geneticists, and genetic counselors elected either not to disclose misattributed paternity or to disclose the information to the mother only.[30,31] Both the confidentiality of the mother and protection of the family unit were cited as reasons for the decision against full disclosure of misattributed paternity.

Although there appears to be agreement among genetic providers toward nondisclosure, many other stakeholders have strongly recommend disclosure of the result to all parties. In fact, nondisclosure or limited disclosure of misattributed paternity appears to be in contrast to ethical concepts of patient autonomy and fidelity. One reason for the discordance between the decision of limited disclosure and promoting patient autonomy may be the definition of the patient. Often, misattributed paternity is identified in a pediatric setting when a child is identified as the patient or in the prenatal setting where the potential mother is identified as the patient. Yet when each partner is counseled about the need for testing, and each partner is consenting to testing, each partner becomes a patient of the genetic provider.[32] The genetic provider would then have an obligation to disclose genetic results to each individual patient.

Furthermore, the decision to disclose results only to the female partner may be in direct conflict with ethical standards. Disclosure to the female partner that the male partner's test was negative (e.g., disclosure that he is not the biological father) is disclosing his results to a third party. The NSGC code of ethics clearly states the obligation to "Maintain information received from clients as confidential, unless released by the client or disclosure is required by law." At the very least the male partner has as much right to his results as any other individual, including the female partner.

Historically, genetic providers have preferred nondisclosure of misattributed paternity due to the possibility that the result would alter the current family dynamics. In this

(*continued*)

situation, clinicians have elected to protect the patient's current social situation rather than risk doing harm by disclosing a potentially disruptive social result. Although the intentions are to limit harm to the patient, it is difficult to balance nonmaleficence and paternalism when making decisions without taking into account the preference of the patient.

Discussing the possibility of misattributed paternity during informed consent is integral to promoting each patient's autonomy. And there may be isolated situations where the appropriate decision is nondisclosure of such sensitive information due to the likelihood of causing harm. Unless there is a case-specific reason or a patient has declared a desire not to know such information during the consent process, the provider should disclose each patient's result and the finding of misattributed paternity to each individual.

BOX 5.2 Case Example: Gaucher Disease

Consider the family depicted in our scenario in which one family member, John, has a known history of Alzheimer disease. His daughter Amy has been concerned about the family history, although she has not decided to pursue testing. Since the birth of her son and the confirmation of her recent pregnancy, Amy has been more concerned about the genetic risk for her children. During one of her early pregnancy-related visits, she discusses all of her concerns with her physician. Her physician attempts to help by referring her to a pulmonologist who is studying the genetic etiology of asthma, a condition that Amy has been treated for since childhood, through exome sequencing. She explains to Amy that the researcher could benefit from another study subject and that Amy may learn of her Alzheimer disease status through the research study.

As Amy's pregnancy progresses she is referred for genetic counseling due to an abnormal multiple marker screen. During the genetic counseling session, Amy reports relief to the genetic counselor that she never heard from the researcher and assumes that meant she was negative for Alzheimer disease. The genetic counselor attempts to explain the limitation of exome sequencing, and that research testing is quite different from clinical testing. Amy is visibly upset and states that she only enrolled in the study to find out what genetic diseases were present that could affect her or her family.

The genetic counselor attends a weekly research update where she happens to sit next to the principal investigator (PI) of the study in which Amy is enrolled. The PI shares her hypothesis that asthma is caused by recessive traits. By examining an autosomal recessive model of inheritance in Amy, the researcher noted that Amy is homozygous for the common Gaucher disease mutation, p.N370S. The PI states that she had no plans to disclose this result to the subject, but since the subject has a relationship with a genetic counselor she would allow the genetic counselor to contact the subject.

The genetic counselor is conflicted. She is not an expert on Gaucher disease, but she does know that only 50% of patients who are homozygous for the p.N370S mutation will develop symptoms of the disease. At the same time, she did not ask Amy questions concerning symptoms of Gaucher disease during the prenatal session, and efficacious treatment in the form of enzyme replacement therapy is readably available.

The genetic counselor is unsure whether she should contact Amy and disclose the result. She appropriately contacts

(*continued*)

her local IRB and discusses the situation. The IRB reviews the study consent form and discusses the study with the PI. Although the consent form does not detail return of results, the IRB recognizes the national recommendations to return those incidental findings that meet criteria of clinical utility and are medically actionable. The IRB leaves the decision of whether this finding meets those criteria to the genetic counselor.

The genetic counselor examines the literature hoping to determine whether Gaucher disease meets existing standards for return of incidental findings. She notes that in one survey of 16 genetic experts, 100% of respondents believed that the finding of Gaucher disease should be disclosed if identified in an adult.[8] But she also noted that Gaucher disease was not included in the recent ACMG recommendations for disclosure of incidental findings.[9] In examining her counseling visit with Amy, the genetic counselor recalls that Amy specifically stated she enrolled in the study with the hope of identifying those genetic results that could impact her health. Disclosing this result would be in agreement with Amy's stated desire for genetic information from the research testing. The genetic counselor also recognizes the possible benefit of identifying a debilitating disease and starting treatment as early as possible. There is the possibility of harm, both by disclosing a result that may never impact Amy's health and by increasing Amy's anxiety, as Amy is already concerned about her risk of Alzheimer disease. The genetic counselor recognizes that providing counseling could minimize the possible harm and arranges a referral to a lysosomal storage expert in a nearby city. She contacts Amy to begin the disclosure process.

Conclusion

The age of personalized medicine is starting to be realized. New technologies have provided access to unprecedented amounts of genetic information, and various entities are poised to interpret it. Soon it may be possible both to identify a patient's genotype and to have a reasonable idea of what that may mean for the individual.

Just as a new paradigm for genomic medicine is starting to emerge, a new model for disclosure of incidental findings must be identified. There are significant differences among genetic providers on the definition of incidental findings, the degree of pretest counseling required before testing, and the best methods of disclosure of incidental findings.[33] Yet most recognize both the importance of disclosure of incidental findings and of appropriate genetic counseling. In a survey of Canadian genomic scientists, most respondents (65%) indicated that genetic counseling should be offered before enrolling in genetic research, and 83% of respondents thought that genetic counseling should be offered before return of research results.[19]

The current model of genetic counseling is easily adaptable to the disclosure of incidental findings. Arguments in favor of disclosure and in favor of nondisclosure both can be persuasive depending on the situation. Protecting patient autonomy is central to genetic counseling, and the types of results that the patient desires should be established during the pretest education and informed-consent process. When an incidental finding is identified, the genetic provider should evaluate both the benefit and possible harm of disclosing the result. Ideally the values of various stakeholders, including researchers, treating physicians, genetic counselors and most importantly the patient, will be factored into the disclosure decision.[19] In general, results that have possible benefits such as early screening, treatment, or reproductive implications should be disclosed to a patient regardless of the context of testing.

REFERENCES

1. Couzin-Frankel, J. (2011). Human genome 10th anniversary. What would you do? *Science*. 331:662–665.
2. Cohen, M.M. Jr. (1971). Variability versus 'incidental findings' in the first and second branchial arch syndrome: unilateral variants with anophthalmia. *Birth Defects Original Articles Series*. 7:103–108.
3. Geelhoed, G.W., Druy, E.M. (1982). Management of the adrenal "incidentaloma." *Surgery*. 92:866–874.
4. Christenhusz, G. M., Devriendt, K., Dierickx, K. (2013). Secondary variants - in defense of a more fitting term in the incidental findings debate. *European Journal of Human Genetics*. 21(12):1331–1334.
5. Anastasova, V., Blasimme, A., Julia, S., Cambon-Thomsen, A. (2013). Genomic incidental findings: reducing the burden to be fair. *American Journal of Bioethics*. 13:52–54.
6. Christenhusz, G.M., Devriendt, K., Dierickx, K. (2013). To tell or not to tell? A systematic review of ethical reflections on incidental findings arising in genetics contexts. *European Journal of Human Genetics*. 21:248–255.
7. Berg, J.S. Adams, M., Nassar, N., Bizon, C., Lee, K., Schmitt, C.P., et al. (2013). An informatics approach to analyzing the incidentalome. *Genetics in Medicine*. 15:36–44.
8. Green, R.C. Berg, J.S., Berry, G.T., Biesecker, L.G., Dimmock, D.P., Evans, J.P., et al. (2012). Exploring concordance and discordance for return of incidental findings from clinical sequencing. *Genetics in Medicine*. 14:405–410.
9. Green, R.C., Berg, J.S., Grody, W.W., Kalia, S.S., Korf, B.R., Martin, C.L. (2013). ACMG recommendations for reporting of incidental findings in clinical exome and genome sequencing. *Genetics in Medicine*. 15(7):565–574.
10. Beauchamp, T.L., Childress, J.F. (2013). *Principles of Biomedical Ethics*. New York: Oxford University Press.
11. Christakis, D.A., Feudtner, C. (1993). Ethics in a short white coat: the ethical dilemmas that medical students confront. *Academic Medicine*. 68:249–254.
12. Fiester, A. (2007). Viewpoint: why the clinical ethics we teach fails patients. *Academic Medicine*. 82:684–689.

13. Caulfield, T., McGuire, A.L., Cho, M., Buchanan, J.A., Burgess, M.M., Danilczyk, U., et al. (2008). Research ethics recommendations for whole-genome research: consensus statement. *PLoS Biology.* 6:e73.
14. Cho, M.K. (2008). Understanding incidental findings in the context of genetics and genomics. *Journal of Law, Medicine, & Ethics.* 36:280–285, 212.
15. Pembrey, M.E., Anionwu, E.N. (1996). Ethical aspects of genetic screening and diagnosis. In D. L. Rimoin, J. M. Connor, R. E. Pyeritz (Eds.). *Emery and Rimoin's principles and practice of medical genetics* (3rd ed.). New York: Churchill Livingstone.
16. Parker, L.S. (2008). The future of incidental findings: should they be viewed as benefits? *Journal of Law, Medicine, &Ethics* 36:341–351, 213.
17. Tabor, H.K., Cho, M.K. (2007). Ethical implications of array comparative genomic hybridization in complex phenotypes: points to consider in research. *Genetics in Medicine.* 9:626–631.
18. Ali-Khan, S.E., Daar, A.S., Shuman, C., Ray, P.N., Scherer, S.W. (2009). Whole genome scanning: resolving clinical diagnosis and management amidst complex data. *Pediatric Research.* 66:357–363.
19. Fernandez, C.V., Strahlendorf, C., Avard, D., Knoppers, B.M., O'Connell, C., Bouffet, E., et al. (2013). Attitudes of Canadian researchers toward the return to participants of incidental and targeted genomic findings obtained in a pediatric research setting. *Genetics in Medicine.* 15(7):558–564.
20. Gliwa, C., Berkman, B.E. (2013). Do researchers have an obligation to actively look for genetic incidental findings? *American Journal of Bioethics.* 13:32–42.
21. National Heart, Lung, and Blood Institute working group, et al. (2010). Ethical and practical guidelines for reporting genetic research results to study participants: updated guidelines from a National Heart, Lung, and Blood Institute working group. *Circulation. Cardiovascular Genetics.* 3:574–580.
22. Canadian Institutes of Health Research, Natural Sciences and Engineering Research Council of Canada & Social Sciences and Humanities Research Council of Canada. (2010). Tri-Council Policy Statement: Ethical Conduct for Research Involving

Humans. Available at http://www.pre.ethics.gc.ca/pdf/eng/tcps2/TCPS_2_FINAL_Web.pdf.

23. Cassa, C. A., Savage, S.K., Taylor, P.L., Green, R.C., McGuire, A.L., Mandl, K.D. (2012). Disclosing pathogenic genetic variants to research participants: quantifying an emerging ethical responsibility. *Genome Research.* 22:421–428.
24. Soderdahl, D. W., Rabah, D., McCune, T., Colonna, J., French, R., Robey, E., et al. (2004). Misattributed paternity in a living related donor: to disclose or not to disclose? *Urology.* 64:590.
25. Wright, L., MacRae, S., Gordon, D., Elliot, E., Dixon, D., Abbey, S., Richardson, R., (2002). Disclosure of misattributed paternity: issues involved in the discovery of unsought information. *Seminars in Dialysis.* 15:202–206.
26. Macintyre, S., Sooman, A. (1991). Non-paternity and prenatal genetic screening. *The Lancet.* 338:869–871.
27. Anderson, K.G. (2006). How well does paternity confidence match actual paternity? Evidence from worldwide nonpaternity rates. *Current Anthropology.* 47:513–520.
28. Andrews, L.B., Fullarton, J.E., Holtzman, N.A., Motulsky, A.G., Eds: Committee on Assessing Genetic Risks, Institute of Medicine. (1994). *Assessing Genetic Risks: Implications for Health and Social Policy.* Washington, DC: The National Academies Press.
29. Lucast, E.K. (2007). Informed consent and the misattributed paternity problem in genetic counseling. *Bioethics.* 21:41–50.
30. Pencarinha, D.F., Bell, N.K., Edwards, J.G., Best, R.G. (1992). Ethical issues in genetic counseling: a comparison of M.S. counselor and medical geneticist perspectives. *Journal of Genetic Counseling.* 1:19–30.
31. Wertz, D.C., Fletcher, J.C., Mulvihill, J.J. (1990). Medical geneticists confront ethical dilemmas: cross-cultural comparisons among 18 nations. *American Journal of Human Genetics.* 46:1200–1213.
32. Ross, L.F. (1996). Disclosing misattributed paternity. *Bioethics.* 10:114–130.
33. Downing, N.R., Williams, J.K., Daack-Hirsch, S., Driessnack, M., Simon, C.M. (2013). Genetics specialists' perspectives on disclosure of genomic incidental findings in the clinical setting. *Patient Education and Counseling.* 90:133–138.

6

Is That a Threat or a Promise? Direct-to-Consumer Marketing of Genetic Testing

LAURA HERCHER

Four weeks to the day after he orders it, an email arrives announcing his "genome scan is complete." Logging into to his account, Peter clicks quickly through the long list of results.

> *Risk of diabetes: neither elevated nor reduced.*
> *Not a carrier for Cystic Fibrosis*
> *Not a carrier for Canavan Disease*—whatever that is.
> *Not a carrier for Sickle Cell Anemia*
> *Male pattern baldness: increased likelihood.*

No surprise there. Peter runs a hand over his close-shaved head, feeling the bristles give way to a smooth expanse across the top.

> *Neanderthal genomic inheritance: 1.7%.*

This seems shockingly high, and yet it is marked in yellow, which means that this result is lower than average. His eyes scan the three-paragraph explanation that accompanies the pie chart, and the picture of a beetle-browed Neanderthal woman holding a stick (or perhaps it is a ladle?), but he soon loses interest and returns to the home screen.

With a sigh, Peter returns to the page marked "list of conditions." Time to get down to business. He finds the entry for Alzheimer disease. It is marked with a little lock icon; this means he must first read a disclaimer and click 'yes' on the box that says "*I understand the potential risks associated with learning about ApoE status and Alzheimer disease. I wish to view my results at this time."* Peter's stomach contracts. His palms are sweaty. He did not expect this, did not expect to feel so nervous. Breathing deeply, he checks the box.

He skips the long description of Alzheimer. He has seen the condition up close, after all. He doesn't need them to tell him what it is like. There is a lot of fine print; he searches through it with increasing impatience. There is so much information here, but it is not what he wants to know—paragraphs on family history, ethnicity, other variants. He scrolls down to the bottom of the page, where it reads:

"Genotype: ApoE e-3, e-2."

But what does that mean? And then below he sees it, the one sentence he has been searching for: "*Your risk of Alzheimer disease is REDUCED relative to the general population.*" Peter exhales deeply and sinks back into his chair. Reduced. The risk is reduced. Slowly his heart rate slows. He reads the sentence a second time, to be sure. "*Your risk of Alzheimer disease is REDUCED relative to the general population.*"

His risk is reduced. But it is not *his* risk. The results on the screen belong to Peter's son Tyler.

For $99 apiece, Peter has ordered genome scans on each of his children. He has not told the kids, and no other family members know anything about this. That way, if the news is bad, he can keep it to himself. Now, if Emma's results match Tyler's, he can stop worrying. And if not, nobody need know—especially not Emma or Tyler.

Direct-to-consumer (or DTC) genetic testing is a relatively new phenomenon. Genome scans, introduced almost simultaneously in a zeitgeist moment in 2007 by Decode Genetics, Navigenics, and 23andMe, have received a great deal of media attention from fans and detractors alike.[1,2] In 2008, the 23andMe scan was *Time*

Magazine's Invention of the Year[3]—while in 2009, *Mother Jones* called their customers "Google's guinea pigs" and insinuated that the company's revenue model was based on selling their customers' genetic information to the pharmaceutical industry and other potential buyers.[4] Although a quick Google search for "genetic testing" will demonstrate that paternity testing is more commonplace, the genome scan is the iconic example of DTC testing and features prominently in the DTC testing debate.

Essentially, the argument over DTC genetic testing focuses on the case for maximizing autonomy and access versus the value of regulation and other methods of protecting consumers. The upside—and the downside—of DTC genetics is that it takes the testing process out of the medical realm and away from medical gatekeepers. This makes it potentially cheaper, more accessible, and in some ways more private. It also permits individuals—or some might say *obligates* individuals—to decide for themselves which tests are worth doing and how to interpret the results. A vocal cohort have made the case that DIY (do it yourself) decision making does not put users at any significant disadvantage given that: (a) a vast amount of information is available online, and (b) there is a woeful lack of genetics expertise among doctors.[5,6,7] To be fair, neither of these observations is in dispute. Nonetheless many medical ethicists, clinicians, and other interested parties, including potential regulators, have expressed concern about the dangers of DTC testing.[8,9,10,11,12,13] Their argument, in essence, is that genetic testing is medical care and that people have reasonable expectations of being protected from practitioners offering medical care that is inappropriate, misleading, useless, or potentially injurious.[14]

DTC genetic testing is posited to put users at risk for various types of harm. One potential negative outcome is that consumers could be scammed. In 2006 the Government Accountability Office (GAO) executed a sting operation on an early version of DTC testing called "nutrigenetics"—an industry based around diet and supplement advice tied to genotype. The GAO report to Congress (subtitled "Tests Purchased from Four Web Sites Mislead Consumers") suggested that the results of nutrigenetic testing were at best without clinical significance and at worst a straight-up con job.[15]

A second type of concern is that tests could have certain legitimacy—that is, they might represent themselves accurately—but that users might misinterpret them, causing consumers to overestimate or underestimate their degree of risk. Overestimates of risk could lead to excessive and inappropriate screening and intervention that was unnecessarily expensive or even dangerous, and underestimates of risk could lead to complacency with inadequate attention paid to preventive medical care or health-modifying behaviors. Concern about scammers suggests that consumers need to be protected from miscreants preying on a vulnerable public and is universally agreed to be as a risk. Concern about misuse of information suggests that consumers need to be protected from themselves and that is a bone of contention among those who criticize the anti-DTC voices as paternalistic.

In general, media reaction to genome scanning has toggled between enthusiasm and skepticism.[16] Other types of DTC genetic tests have received a similar love-it-or-hate-it reception. An online dating service making the claim that their matches were based on DNA was ridiculed by experts, while simultaneously being the subject of cheerful, enthusiastic features on ABC News, the *Washington Post,* and the Huffington Post.[17,18,19] The Atlas Genetics "SportsGene" test for "athletic advantage" was derided by the academic community, including the geneticist on whose work the claims were based,[20] but received largely uncritical press from the *New York Times* in its article "Born to Run? Little Ones Get Test for Sports Gene." The article did strike a single obligatory cautionary note: "Some . . . say $ACTN_3$ testing is in its infancy and virtually useless . . ."—but only in paragraph eight.[21]

Amid the general themes of fascination and disdain, a number of distinct lines of criticism have emerged. Three questions in particular have dominated the conversation:

1. Are DTC results accurate; namely, is the lab work reliable?
2. Are the tests offered DTC clinically meaningful, and can they be understood without the help of medical experts?
3. Is DTC testing more subject to abuse, such as privacy violations or the exploitation of vulnerable individuals?

First, there are concerns regarding the reliability of the testing process itself, which is a question of lab quality. Medical testing, by law, is done only in labs supervised by the Centers for Medicare and Medicaid through CLIA (the Clinical Laboratories Improvement Amendments), which is charged with ensuring lab standards. The 2006 GAO report on nutrigenetics was scathing—but it acknowledged that all blank samples sent in, as well as those from cats or dogs, came back labeled "impossible to process." While critical, the government assessment suggested that in these early incarnations of the DTC model, analytic validity (lab accuracy) was better than clinical validity (meaningfulness).[15]

Still, as the industry moves toward greater potential diagnostic and health-related significance, the importance of CLIA certification as a consumer protection issue has increased. Nonmedical testing can be done in a non-CLIA lab, which saves money; medical testing cannot. Naturally, the DTC companies have been resistant to describing their tests as "medical," since that would invite intrusive and expensive government regulation. Health reports from 23andMe come with a disclaimer at the bottom that reads, "*The genotyping services of 23andMe are performed in LabCorp's CLIA-certified laboratory. The tests have not been cleared or approved by the FDA but have been analytically validated according to CLIA standards. The information on this page is intended for research and educational purposes only, and is not for diagnostic use.*" At the same time, the selling point of these tests for susceptibility to cancer, heart disease, and macular degeneration is clinical significance (or at least it was until the FDA ordered them to halt sales of its genetic tests in late 2013 because they had not received regulatory clearance). Over the years, this tension has been apparent in the marketing strategies for genome scans, which are routinely touted as an opportunity to invest in your own health ("*Living well starts with knowing your DNA.*") but deliver results marked "*not for diagnostic use.*"[22]

Regulatory zeal regarding the need for CLIA certification has varied by state. In 2008, New York and California sent letters to companies offering DTC genome scanning requiring them to cease and desist testing without certification.[23] New York and California singled out genome scans because they purported to have medical implications; other forms of testing have drawn less scrutiny. Peter, our concerned father, used a scan from 23andMe—the only one of the original DTC genome scans still on the market in 2013. He could have read the section on "Technology and Standards" and seen that "*All of the laboratory testing for 23andMe is done in a CLIA-certified laboratory.*"[22] But like most people, Peter skipped the technical stuff, assuming that 23andMe, which he had read about in the *New York Times*, must have a reliable laboratory. If they were not legitimate, he reasoned, the government would shut them down. There are laws against frauds and hucksters.

The second question, the one about meaning, while perhaps not more significant is clearly more difficult to answer. Are the results meaningful? There are a number of ways to judge. One is to measure the **reliability** of the association between genotype and phenotype: an assessment of how well documented the association between the gene and the condition or disease is. Has it been replicated? Have the studies looked at a big enough sample to rule out randomness? Has it been demonstrated in a variety of ethnic groups or only a single, genetically homogeneous population? If the answer to any of these questions is no, the relationship between the gene and the outcome must be considered speculative.

A second test is to look at the **strength** of the association. Do studies suggest that this gene variant actually moves the dial on the likelihood of disease? Many studies of genetic risk produce reliable results with tiny effect sizes. For example, one variant that is a part of the 23andMe panel for type II diabetes risk has an odds ratio of 1.03, which means that if your prior presumed risk for diabetes was 10%, your adjusted risk after finding out you carried this variant (in round numbers) is: still 10%. In fact, tiny effect sizes are the rule and not the exception in studies of common variants contributing to genetic proclivity for disease. These results may be very interesting to a researcher because they say something about the cause or natural history of the disease; but they are not informative for an individual looking for information with health implications, and their inclusion can be misleading. Some algorithms look at many variants associated with a given condition and sum them up for a total risk score that theoretically has more power. However, there is no reason to assume that individual associations are additive and many reasons to assume that they are not. Most traits associated with common complex disease do not have simple, quantitative measures of risk that add up. The underlying genetic risks may reflect diverse pathways that are essentially unrelated to one another—genes that do not have interacting effects—or gene-to-gene interactions (epistatic effects) that are much more complicated than one plus one equals two.

Peter's search for Alzheimer risk status presents a good example of risk analysis in a trait where the genetic factors are not quantitative. The result he is looking at, for ApoE genotype, is an important risk factor with real implications: it is a reliable and well-documented association with significant predictive value. But his father's genetic predisposition to Alzheimer is based on a different gene, one that is rarer and leads to early-onset dementia rather than garden variety late-in-life disease. The disease looks the same but the mechanism is quite different.

In each case, dementia is caused by a build-up of a harmful protein product in the brain. ApoE subtype affects the body's ability to clear away this protein more efficiently, so that a build-up occurs over time. John, Peter's father, had a presenilin mutation that directly affected the amount and toxicity of the protein product produced in the brain—in cases such as this, the disease will present regardless of the body's housekeeping abilities, so that the ApoE risk factor is moot.

A third way to inquire about meaningfulness is to ask whether the outcome of the test will have any real-life **importance** for the recipient. There are a number of ways to measure this as well. Some test results may alter medical care. Results can suggest a need for a different treatment, a change in the type or dosage of medication, or preventive measures like high-risk screening. Test results with the potential to alter medical care are referred to as "clinically actionable." Of course, genetic testing may have an impact outside of the clinical setting as well. Advocates for genetic screening have suggested that people will find their genetic test results an impetus to improve health-related behaviors associated with the conditions for which they have increased risk, and some small and preliminary studies have documented modest positive effects.[24] The potential for genetic tests to have the opposite effect—to negatively impact health-related behavior out of complacency or fatalism—has not been studied.

Frequently these debates revolve around conditions where "improved health-related behavior" includes only garden-variety, commonsensical moves that are likely to be beneficial in any event: don't smoke, eat more vegetables, maintain a healthy body weight, exercise regularly, and so on. The stakes are lower when the advice all falls into the category of "it can't hurt." Yet another way to judge meaningfulness is to establish categories of risk that are by definition not garden-variety. Test results that indicate a risk with **serious implications that are not routine**—a risk that suggests the need for intervention that is not generic—establish a different sort of obligation on the part of whoever orders or does the testing. For example, BRCA 1 and 2 testing, in which positive results can lead to prophylactic removal of the breasts and ovaries, may require more oversight and create obligations of care similar to a traditional doctor–patient relationship. This is qualitatively different from testing for a gene where those who test positive are urged to substitute olive oil for butter or take a multivitamin daily.

Similarly, test results that lay bare a potential harm that the individual would have had no way to anticipate in the absence of testing bring with them serious concomitant responsibilities. Genetic tests may identify individuals at increased risk for smoking-related morbidity and mortality, and while this is very important and useful information it is safe to assume that consumers already know that smoking is a threat to their health. In comparison, pharmacogenetic tests indicating an equally serious but much rarer risk—a predisposition to a certain side effect, for example, or a metabolic irregularity that could affect response to anesthesia—will potentially alert an individual to a significant and unknown danger. Failing to deliver or mishandling this sort of game-changing information could have the type of consequences we associate with inadequate or incompetent medical care—and may require similar forms of regulation and redress.

While some measures of meaningfulness look to find whether an association between a gene and a condition has any significance at all, this final standard looks to find if the value of the test is not only real but **compels action**. Failures of the first type—like inadequacies in the strength or the reliability of the association—may be misleading even if the information as reported is technically accurate and given in good faith (and the fact that it might not be done in good faith should come as no surprise to anyone using the Internet, so buyer beware). Gross violations deemed a significant enough threat to the public can be addressed through existing consumer protection entities such as the Federal Trade Commission, which safeguards consumers against false advertising. But what about the last? What about the highly consequential health-related information that compels actions under what we might think of as a duty-to-warn standard? Can that information be given out, without access to medical help, without inviting adverse consequences?

After all, the question of whether a genetic test can be considered meaningful is equally complex in a clinical or DTC setting. The only issue specific to DTC is the absence or potential absence of whatever help medical caregivers might offer in making that determination. This "help" is portrayed very differently by advocates on either side. Those in favor of regulation highlight the importance of medical expertise and objective advice. Proponents of DTC testing question both the value and the objectivity of medical caregivers, and many see a built-in institutional bias toward maintaining control of the infrastructure of medical testing. "BREAKING: gatekeepers opposed to open gates" tweeted Daniel MacArthur of the Broad Institute, in response to an article documenting clinical geneticists' continued opposition to DTC testing.[25]

Let's consider what might medical assistance have done for Peter. The information available on the 23andMe website accurately describes the impact of the ApoE genotype on Alzheimer disease risk assessment. But although Peter is educated and intelligent and easily comprehends the material as presented, his understanding of the true dynamics of the situation is fundamentally flawed. His sister Amy might have told him that in their father's case, ApoE status is irrelevant. But Peter's plan revolved around secrecy, so he did not reveal his decision to test, and therefore the conversation with Amy that might have ensued did not. Someone else might have done a more thorough job researching the matter online. The likelihood of this happening is a function of both education and personality. Peter—like many people—avoided immersing himself in a subject that was so viscerally distressing. As proponents of DTC testing have pointed out, the amount of information available online is enormous. As critics of DTC testing have pointed out, the subject matter is complex and the potential for misunderstanding is great.

Would the participation of a medical professional have helped? In other circumstances it might not have been necessary. Peter's family could have explained the situation to him after the testing was done on his father. Why didn't they? In this case, not telling Peter was his mother's idea. Amy was contemplating another pregnancy, but Peter was not—what good would it do him to know? "Say nothing to your brother," she said.

In Peter's case, a genetics professional would have alerted him to his misreading of the situation and, should he have desired it, directed him toward more appropriate testing for himself. At the same time, most genetic counselors or geneticists would have balked at testing the children in accordance with widely followed practice standards that advise against testing children for adult-onset conditions that cannot be prevented (see chapter 4).[26,27,28] As a rule, individuals in the field consider testing minors to be unethical, since it is potentially stigmatizing and takes away the child's right to make the choice for him or herself as an adult. So had Peter sought help, he would likely have gotten a clearer understanding of the facts but no assistance in getting the tests done. Does this constitute help or obstructionism? Paternalism or protection of the children? Passions run high on both sides.[29]

Without suggesting that it is simple to find a balance between protection and access, two generalizations can be made. First, this information has an increasing amount of medical significance and therefore entails a fairly high level of vigilance. Truth in advertising is the province of the Federal Trade Commission, which is constrained by budget and manpower restrictions and must pick its battles. They can be expected to go after misrepresentations that are egregious or clearly dangerous; making other sources of truth-checking available would be good for both consumers and the field of genetics, which risks being tainted by bad practices and misleading test results. Second, as a rule, restricting access to information is the more globally undesirable outcome since an overabundance of information can be refined over time into something more useful, while restrictions produce no opportunities for accumulated wisdom. If that wisdom is to be accumulated at some cost to certain individuals, then we have to question how steep a cost we can, in fairness, accommodate.

What level of oversight do the users of DTC testing services desire? **They want to be protected, and they want autonomy**. A survey of DTC customers published in 2013 illustrates the conflict: 84% of the 1046 respondents preferred to have a governmental or nongovernmental agency ensure that claims made by DTC companies were consistent with scientific evidence, but two-thirds of the same group indicated that it was "important that DTC tests be available without governmental oversight."[30] Obviously, finding the optimal balance between providing some assurances to consumers and removing barriers to access will be no easy task.

The idea that regulation might impede the ability of an individual to get information available through genetic testing without going through medical intermediaries is offensive to many, who view it as an infringement of users' rights and authority.[31] Currently, sans regulation, there are neither impediments nor obligations: in theory, consumers can get any test they want but with no guarantee that they are getting accurate, complete, or medically significant information. Some DTC companies are incentivized to be trustworthy—trustworthiness might be an article of faith or a part of their long-term business plan—but others are not. In 2011, a company called My Gene Profile (now reborn as "Map *my* Gene") offered one test billed as "your complete disease susceptibility genetic test" for $1897 and another, similarly priced, to profile "your child's talent genes and personality genes." "*What if you are told your child could be the next Einstein, Bill Gates or the next Tiger Woods...*" boomed the advertisement. While this level of hyperbole might make it easier to tell the wheat from the chaff, judging true credibility remains a complicated research project even for the most science-literate.

Perhaps in response to this and similar assaults on the respectability of their nascent industry, 23andMe reversed a long-standing resistance to FDA regulation in 2012 and actually requested that the agency weigh in on several of its tests.[32] This extraordinary step capped a transformation of the DTC landscape that had occurred in the 2 years since the FDA first asserted its intent to regulate DTC testing.[33]

Five companies received letters from the FDA in May 2010: 23andMe, deCode Genetics, Knome, Navigenics and Illumina. At the time, all except Illumina were offering a form of genome scanning available for purchase online; Illumina provided the chips for all of the companies involved. The services themselves varied dramatically. Navigenics, DeCode Genetics, and 23andMe each offered a test based on a custom-designed chip that allowed them to look at thousands of individual markers throughout the genome. Although their techniques were similar, their approaches were different: Navigenics focused on what they viewed as medically relevant results with clinical significance, while 23andMe invited customers to consider both the serious and the frivolous implications of their genetic makeup—they included reports on ancestry and information on variants with little or no relationship to health, such as the propensity to hair loss or the quality of one's ear wax. Occupying the middle ground was the test from DeCode Genetics, which offered a wider range of information than Navigenics but maintained an emphasis on health-related results, albeit at a higher price point than either of its competitors. For price, however, the clear outlier was Knome, which offered not a scan but a full genome sequence—at a cost of $68,500. A relative bargain, since Knome's first customers in 2008 had paid $350,000 apiece.

Some implications of the FDA action were immediate. Pathway Genomics, which had announced a plan to sell its test kit in all Walgreens stores only weeks before the letters arrived, suspended and then cancelled its in-store operation and ultimately withdrew from the DTC market altogether. Similarly, Navigenics ended online sales in 2010, choosing instead to market its genome-based risk assessment as a clinical resource. The Iceland-based company DeCode Genetics, struggling for survival in the aftermath of the 2008 financial collapse, was sold to Amgen in December 2012, and the DeCodeMe genomic scan was discontinued.

The DTC testing industry has experienced considerable upheaval since the FDA letters went out in 2010, but none of it can be traced to a tightening of regulatory control because until recently no regulation or clarification of regulatory intent has actually been produced. The inherent difficulty of establishing or policing a standard for what constitutes reliability and meaning beyond basic measures of technical competence has proved too much of a stumbling block, and that is yet another reason to be leery of government regulation as a solution to the problems caused by DTC testing. A compromise position might be to focus on providing independent resources for decision making and fact checking that could give DTC customers the opportunity to make better choices and put test results in context. Another possible approach—and these are not mutually exclusive—would be to focus on identifying a narrowly drawn subset of tests where the results compel action, and use this designation to single out tests that require the attention of regulators.

Separating reliable from less reliable forms of DTC testing has already been an issue for tests with legal significance. Paternity tests, for example, may be done two ways, and both are available DTC. The cheaper option, from a laboratory that may or may not have CLIA certification, uses DNA samples sent in by the customer. The second, which is admissible in court, uses a certified facility and maintains chain of custody to assure the identity of the individuals tested.

While medical significance is different than legal significance, there are certain parallels. Customers using DTC genetic testing are frequently encouraged by the testing companies to share their results with their healthcare providers. When they do, the job of establishing analytic and clinical validity is a problem passed along from the DTC company to the medical professional. The doctor, nurse, or counselor must then decide which part of these reports should be looked at carefully and which should be dismissed out of hand. Is a caregiver responsible for interpreting the results of a test he or she did not order? Is it reasonable to use the test results from the DTC laboratory, or does the test need to be redone? While some poking around may enable the clinician to find out whether the source is reliable (or at minimum, CLIA certified), in general it is safest for them to treat DTC information as analogous to other forms of patient-generated data, like a family history or oral reports of medical history—which means, from the point of view of the medical professional, trust but verify.

A final topic that fuels the DTC debate is the issue of vulnerability to fraud and the loss of privacy. Obviously fraud did not begin with the invention of the Internet. One reason for regulation of medical practice and treatments in general is the universal acknowledgment that individuals facing sickness or death have a special vulnerability (and that there are and always have been unscrupulous people willing to prey on that vulnerability). In this sense, autonomy or no autonomy, all patients are routinely protected from their own susceptibility to the lure of miracles. The key word here is *patients*: outside of what we define as medical practice, you are free to throw your money away as you see fit.

Is DTC genetic testing the practice of medicine? To date the absence of regulation suggests that it is not, but other assessments place it in a gray area.[14] Like vitamins or massage therapy, it is a health-related product that consumers negotiate on their own. Overselling the value or accuracy of testing ("What if you are told your child could be the next Einstein, Bill Gates or the next Tiger Woods...?") is a problem that can sometimes be addressed through market-based corrections. In 2005, Acu-Gen rolled out its Baby Gender Mentor test with a debut on the *Today Show*. The test, which looked for traces of Y-chromosome DNA in the maternal bloodstream, claimed to be 99.9% accurate in determining fetal gender. Although the method was sound, the sensitivity fell below 99%, and the company was forced to withdraw their product after complaints from a number of unhappy mothers who gave birth to children of the "wrong" gender. The company filed for Chapter 11 bankruptcy protection in 2009.

There is a blurry line between hype and fraud, and many DTC genetic testing products have tested the distinction. The 2006 GAO report on DTC sales of nutrigenetic testing cast doubt on the legitimacy of the field as a whole, calling the results of testing "medically unproven and so ambiguous that they do not provide meaningful information to consumers." What's more, two of the companies attempted to capitalize on the spurious testing data to sell their customers vitamins tailored to their "unique" genetic profile. A 1-year supply of "personalized nutritional formula" from one website cost $1200; the GAO determined that the supplements contained nothing that could not be obtained from a typical multivitamin and put the retail value at $35 per year.[15] A second GAO investigation of DTC genetic testing companies in 2010 found many irregularities in how the scans were marketed, including the widely publicized fact that in certain instances GAO employees posing as customers were encouraged to send in samples on behalf of a fiancé without that individual's knowledge or consent.[34]

Still, while problematic, this is garden-variety fraud and not a phenomenon uniquely tied to the field of genetics. Should consumers need assistance to determine that a test for their warrior roots—described as "a full and accurate historical profile on your ancient ancestors..."—is not a reliable source of family history?[35] What about "the warrior gene" as featured on the *Dr. Phil* television show and the National Geographic Channel documentary "Explorer: Born to Rage?" The so-called warrior gene—a variant of an MAO inhibitor linked to increased aggression in response to provocation—has more credibility, and therefore more real-world implications, which perhaps makes it more and not less of a risk for consumers.[36,37,38] Still, no mechanism exists or should exist under which it would be possible to limit dissemination of this information via the Internet.

Arguably, in these cases the risk is not in the testing itself but in the gullibility of a customer primed to believe in a simple narrative of genetic determinism.

Privacy concerns, on the other hand, are uniquely tied to genetics and cannot be addressed through education or market-driven correctives. There are a number of privacy-related issues. Some concerns involve putting DNA samples linked to names, and at times health information or other personal details, into the hands of private companies. There is no question that the market for genetic information exists and is likely to expand. Pharmaceutical companies and researchers are motivated to obtain DNA data linked to health outcomes. Several recent examples suggest a developing interest among marketing and retail entities in genetic information linked to names and demographics.[39,40] In the business world there is no single standard for privacy policies. Analysts have suggested that commercial use of their database is integral to the 23andMe long-term financial plan,[41] an assertion backed up by public statements from 23andMe executives and board members.[42] Their privacy policy does not constrain their use of information gleaned from genome scans and associated questionnaires on health history, which the company claims are filled out by nearly 90% of all 23andMe customers.[43]

Of course, to say that the information will be used is not to say that it will be used for nefarious purposes. Many 23andMe customers might be pleased to find that their genetic information was being used for the study of disease and wellness. An emphasis on the negative reflects little in the way of specific present harms and more a fear of what is unknown and potentially unforeseen. And 23andMe is only one example of a company collecting genomic data and may not be representative in its emphasis on research and community building.

Company policies regarding the use of genetic information obtained through DTC sources may be shaped over time by consumer sentiment and experience. Less amenable to market pressure is the wealth of DNA data available online that is not under corporate control. Ancestry sites as well as DTC genetics companies focusing on ancestry routinely facilitate sharing snippets of DNA in publicly accessible databases, which permit people with shared ancestry to locate one another. Stories of family members reunited have generally received media attention as a positive phenomenon.[44,45,46] Some sites specialize in reuniting adopted children and biological relatives as well as long-lost cousins and so on. While the presumption is that anyone making their DNA results available is open to being contacted, it is not such an easy process to control given that DNA matches from other biological relatives can easily suggest the identity of parents, children, siblings, and the like.[47] The reverse it also true: DNA-sharing sites may also reveal nonrelatedness between presumptive biological family members, a specter familiar to anyone working in clinical genetics.

The ever-increasing amount of DNA available online has other implications as well. There is a growing debate over the appropriate use of DNA databases in forensic cases. While those with the most to hide might be clever enough to avoid posting their own DNA to accessible sites, to be safe they would need to control the actions of all close relatives. The issue around using DNA in this manner concerns mainly our ability to assure that matches made strictly based on genetic code are accurate. A recent study suggests that forensic use of DNA databases is an accurate way to identify persons of interest, with some caveats. In general, the technology correctly identified individuals and their relatives. The important note of caution from this study was that distant relatives were at times misidentified as close relatives, while the reverse was never true.[48]

Public availability of DNA samples linked to names also affects the privacy of research participants. Promising anonymity to research subjects has been commonplace and has smoothed the way for data sharing, which is an increasingly important practice in the genomic age where large datasets are often necessary to provide meaningful results. A number of recent studies have cast doubt on the ability of researchers to provide anonymity simply by removing names, in light of the public DNA databases and the innate power of DNA as a potent identifier. In 2013, Whitehead Institute fellow Yaniv Erlich and others published an account in *Science* describing the use of short tandem repeats on the Y chromosome and publicly available information to identify research participants whose DNA sequences were available anonymously online.[49] While Erlich shared the names only with authorities at the National Human Genome Research Institute (NHGRI), his proof-in-principle experiment made the point quite dramatically that the days of achieving anonymity for DNA data are gone. "We are in what I call an awareness moment," said Eric Green of NHGRI, responding to news of what Erlich had accomplished using tools no more powerful than a decent Internet connection.[50]

What these and other privacy-busting experiments have shown is that controlling how corporations or researchers use DNA data is inadequate to ensure that the sequences are not identifiable, since the voluntary publishing of DNA data compromises privacy for not only the individuals who make that choice but also their immediate—and not so immediate—family members. Like researchers, DTC companies will have to be mindful of these new realities and craft consents and other documentation that reflect the restrictions on anonymity and the consequences of public sharing of DNA sequence information.

For Peter, his foray into genetic testing had no disastrous effects but fell short of what he had hoped it could achieve. It was, as Anders Nordgren described DTC risk prediction in a 2012 article in the *Journal of Community Genetics*, "neither as harmful as feared by critics nor as empowering as promised by providers."[51] By consensus this is a decent summary of our collective experience with DTC genetics in its first decade. Its future as an adjunct or a replacement for clinical uses of genetic testing remains to be seen, and while the potential benefits provide a reason to move forward we must move forward with care and vigilance—care, and vigilance, and an open mind.

REFERENCES

1. Caulfield, T., Mcguire, A.L. (2012). Direct-to-consumer genetic testing: perceptions, problems and policy responses. *Annual Review of Medicine*. 63:22–23.
2. Rahm, A.K., Deering, J., Feigelson, H.S., Tracer, D., Bull, S. (2011). Media messages and public perception of direct-to-consumer genetics: result of a media analysis and focus group study. *Clinical Medicine and Research*. 9(3–4):177.
3. Hamilton, A. (2008). Invention of the year: the retail DNA test. *Time Magazine*. October 29, 2008.
4. Brownlee, S. (2009). Google's Guinea Pigs (data mining your DNA). *Mother Jones*. Nov 11, 2009.
5. Vayena, E., Prainsack, B. (2013). Regulating genomics: time for a broader vision. *Science Translational Medicine*. 5(198):198.
6. MacArthur, D. (2011). American Medical Association: you can't look at your genome without our supervision. *Wired Science blogs, Genetic Future* Feb 24 2011. Available at: http://www.wired.com/wiredscience/2011/02/american-medical-association-you-cant-look-at-your-genome-without-our-supervision/.
7. Angrist, M. (2009). We are the genes we have been waiting for: rational responses to the gathering storm of personal genomics. *American Journal of Bioethics*. 9(6–7):30–31.
8. ACMG Statement on Direct-to-Consumer Genetic Testing, American College of Medicine Genetics Board of Directors, January/February 2004.
9. Wasson, K., Cook, E.D., Helzlsouer, K. (2006). Direct-to-consumer online genetic testing and the four principles: an analysis of the ethical issues. *Ethics in Medicine*. 22(2):8–91.
10. American Society of Human Genetics. (2007). Statement on direct-to-consumer genetic testing in the United States. *American Journal of Human Genetics*. 81:635–637.
11. Vorhaus, D. (2010). "From Gulf Oil to Snake Oil": Congress Takes Aim at DTC Genetic Testing" *Genomics Law Report*, July 22, 2010. Available at: http://www.genomicslawreport.com/index.php/2010/07/22/from-gulf-oil-to-snake-oil-congress-takes-aim-at-dtc-genetic-testing/.
12. European Society of Human Genetics. (2010). Statement of the ESHG on direct-to-consumer genetic testing for health-related purposes. *European Journal of Human Genetics*. 1–3.

13. Howard, H.C., Borry, P. (2013). Survey of European clinical geneticists on awareness, experiences and attitudes towards direct-to-consumer genetic testing. *Genome Medicine* 5:45.
14. Marietta, C., Maguire, A.L. (2009). Direct-to-consumer genetic testing: is it the practice of medicine? *Journal of Law and Medical Ethics*. 37(2):369–374.
15. Government Accountability Office. (2006). "Nutrigenetic testing: tests purchased from four websites mislead customers." Testimony before the Special Committee on Aging, U.S. Senate, July 27, 2006.
16. Lynch, J., Parrott, A., Hopkin, R.A., Myers, M. (2011). Media coverage of direct-to-consumer genetic testing. *Journal of Genetic Counseling*. 5:486–494.
17. Friedman, E. (2007). Can DNA tests help find true love? *ABC News*, Dec 13, 2007. Available at: http://abcnews.go.com/Health/story?id=3991467&page=1#.UYKcG79vUml.
18. Scott, M. (2009). ScientificMatch.com uses DNA samples to make perfect couple. *HuffPost Style*, Nov 12, 2009. Available at: http://www.huffingtonpost.com/2009/11/13/scientificmatchcom-uses-d_n_356646.html.
19. McCarthy, E. (2010). To link singles, matchmaker dives into the gene pool. *The Washington Post*, Jan 24, 2010.
20. MacArthur, D. (2008). The ACTN3 sports gene test: what can it really tell you? *Genetic Future at Wired.com*, Nov. 30, 2008.
21. Macur, J. (2008). Born to run: little ones get test for sports gene. *The New York Times*, Nov 29, 2008.
22. 23andMe website, October 2, 2013. See: https://www.23andme.com/health/
23. Kaye, J. (2008). The regulation of direct-to-consumer genetic tests. *Human Molecular Genetics*. 17(r2):180–183.
24. Kaufman, D.J., Bollinger, J.M., Dvoskin, R.L., Scott, J.A. (2012). Risky business: risk perception and the use of medical services among customers of DTC personal genetic testing. *Journal of Genetic Counseling*. 21(3):413–422.
25. MacArthur, D. (dgmacarthur). "BREAKING: gatekeepers opposed to open gates. RT @C_G_S: Clinical geneticists opposed to DTC genetic testing bit.ly/13DdDp5." June 4, 2013 4:26 PM. Tweet.
26. American Academy of Pediatrics, American College of Medical Genetics and Genomics. (2013). Ethical and policy issues in genetic testing and screening of children. *Pediatrics*. 131:620–622.

27. Ross, L.F., Saal, H.M., David, K.L., Anderson, R.R. American Academy of Pediatrics; American College of Medical Genetics and Genomics. (2013). Technical report: ethical and policy issues in genetic testing and screening of children. *Genetics in Medicine.* 15(3):234–245.
28. National Society of Genetic Counselors: Position Statement on Genetic Testing of Minors for Adult-Onset Conditions, adopted 2012.
29. Evans, J.P., Green, R.C. (2009). Direct-to-consumer genetic testing: Avoiding a culture war. *Genetic in Medicine.* 11(8): 568–569.
30. Bollinger, J.M., Green, R.C., Kaufman, D. (2013). Attitudes about regulation among direct-to-consumer genetic testing customers. *Genetic Testing and Molecular Biomarkers.* 17(5):424–428.
31. Kahn, R. (2011). Your genes, your rights—FDA's Jeffrey Shuren misleading testimony under oath. *Discover blogs: Gene Expression.* March 9, 2011. Available at: http://blogs.discovermagazine.com/gnxp/2011/03/your-genes-your-rights-fdas-jeffrey-shuren-not-a-fan/#.Uk2aUBZsZgs.
32. Perrone, M. (2012). 23andMe seeks FDA approval for personal DNA test. *Businessweek*, July 30, 2012.
33. Shuren, J. (2012). Direct-to-Consumer Genetic Testing and the Consequences to the Public Testimony to the Subcommittee on Oversight and Investigations, Committee on Energy and Commerce, U.S. House of Representatives, July 22, 2010.
34. Kutz, G. (2010). Direct-to-consumer genetic tests: misleading test results are further complicated by deceptive marketing and other questionable practices. Congressional Testimony. July 22, 2010.
35. Warrior Roots. Website, Oct 7, 2013. Available at: http://www.warriorroots.com/warrior.html
36. Dr. Phil: Born to rage? July 26, 2011. See: http://www.drphil.com/shows/show/1626
37. National Geographic Channel: Inside the Warrior Gene. December 14, 2010. See: http://natgeotv.com.au/tv/inside-the-warrior-gene/
38. McDermott, R., Tingley, D., Cowden, J., Frazzetto, G., Johnson, D.D. (2008). Monoamine oxidase A gene (MAOA) predicts behavioral aggression following provocation. *Proceedings of*

the National Academy of Sciences of the United States of America. 106(7):2118–2123.

39. Abraham, C. (2012). Why your DNA is a goldmine for marketers. *The Globe and Mail*, December 12, 2012.
40. Hernandez D (2013). Selling your most personal item: you. *Wired*, March 27, 2013. Available at: http://www.wired.com/business/2013/03/miinome-genetic-marketplace/.
41. Vorhaus, D. (2012). As DeCODE departs, 23andMe reloads. *Genomics Law Report*. December 11, 2012. Available at: http://www.genomicslawreport.com/index.php/tag/23andme/
42. Murphy, E. (2013). Inside 23andMe founder and CEO Anne Wojcicki's $99 DNA Revolution. *Fast Company*, October 14, 2013. Available at: http://www.fastcompany.com/3018598/for-99-this-ceo-can-tell-you-what-might-kill-you-inside-23andme-founder-anne-wojcickis-dna-r
43. 23andMe. (2012). Press release, December 20: 23andMe Presents Top Ten Most Interesting Genetic findings of 2012. Available at: http://www.prnewswire.com/news-releases/23andme-presents-top-ten-most-interesting-genetic-findings-of-2012-184273541.html.
44. Swarns, R.L. (2012). With DNA testing, suddenly they are family. *New York Times*, January 23, 2012.
45. CNN: 23andMe and search angel reunite mother and son. February 1, 2013. Available at: http://ireport.cnn.com/docs/DOC-918630.
46. Steve Harvey Show: Father & Daughter Reunion, September 3, 2013. Available at: http://steveharveytv.com/father-daughter-reunion/
47. Hill, K. (2012). Whoops. How DNA Site 23andMe outed parents who gave up their baby for adoption. *Forbes*, May 16 2012. Available at: http://www.forbes.com/sites/kashmirhill/2012/05/16/dna-site-23andme-outed-parents-who-gave-their-first-baby-up-for-adoption/.
48. Rohlfs, R.V., Murphy, E., Song, Y.S., Slatkin, M. (2013). The influence of relatives on the efficiency and error rate of familial searching. *PLoS One*. 8(8):e70495.
49. Gymrek, M., McGuire, A.L., Golan, D., Halperin, E., Erlich, Y. (2013). Identifying personal genomes by surname inference. *Science*. 339:321–324.

50. Kolata, G. (2013). Web hunt for DNA sequences leaves privacy compromised. *New York Times*, January 17, 2013.
51. Nordgren, A. (2012). Neither as harmful as feared by critics nor as empowering as promised by providers: risk information offered direct to consumer by personal genomics companies. *Journal of Community Genetics (EPub).*

7

Genetics and Patent Law

REBECCA R. ANDERSON

We join Amy, Joy, Michael and Peter as a mild summer evening draws to a close. The kids are playing in the backyard as the adults sit around the remains of a campfire.

Peter: So, Michael, why are we hearing so much in the news about gene patents?

Michael: Are you sure you want to get me started on this?

Joy: Why not? We can always take a nap if you get too boring.

Michael: Okay, settle in for your bedtime story. Once upon a time, there were three kinds of patents: design patents, plant patents, and utility patents.

Design patents[1] let you protect the aesthetic elements of a manufactured article. But they've never been very popular because for a lot of things you can get longer and better and cheaper protection under trademark or copyright law—like when you copyright stamp your pottery, Joy.

Joy: Right.

Michael: Plant patents[2] let you protect new varieties you've developed. You can even patent plants you find growing wild, so long as you first bring them under cultivation. But you can only get a plant patent on plants that can be reproduced asexually—like cuttings or divisions or grafting. Plant patents aren't allowed on seed-grown plants.

Amy: How come?

Michael: Two reasons, as I recall. One is that with tissue culture you can be pretty sure the daughter plant is identical to the parent plant. They are essentially clones. But with seed-grown plants there is a good chance the next generation won't run true and will no longer be the same plant for which you got the patent.

The other reason is that when Congress set up this system in 1930, it decided it would be a bad idea to give people monopolies on major food crops. Oh—and you couldn't patent tuber-grown plants like potatoes, for the same reason.

Amy: But what about Monsanto's soybeans?

Michael: Hang on; that part of the story comes later. We have to build up some suspense first.

Now, the Papa Bear of the patent family is the utility patent.[3] Utility patents let you protect mechanical inventions, manufacturing and processing methods, new chemicals and compounds—all the stuff you usually think of when you think of patents.

To get one of these patents, your invention has to satisfy three criteria: it has to be novel,[4] useful, and non-obvious.[5] "Novel" means that it's distinctively different from existing technology: nobody else was making or using it before you invented it; nobody else already applied for a patent on the same thing. "Useful" means it has some benefit for society. And "non-obvious" means that it isn't something any idiot could have come up with. Actually, it means that the invention isn't obvious to someone with "ordinary skill in the art." So if I were claiming a new way of making shoes, I'd be held to an obviousness standard among shoemakers.

You also have to describe in detail all the elements of your invention—that's called the "enablement." Essentially, you disclose all of the steps of making and using your invention so that anyone reasonably skilled in the art would be able to make and use it. And you have to write "claims" that tell exactly what you're staking out as your patented territory, so that other people in the business can figure out what the boundaries are. Your claims have to be supported by your disclosure, and they can't infringe on anyone else's claims from previous patents.

So the trade-off you make when you get a patent is that you disclose your invention to the world, and in return you get to keep anyone else from using it for a set number of years.

Peter: How long?

Michael: For utility patents it's 20 years now, from the date of filing.

Peter: Hence the monopoly.

Michael: Yes, but notice that your patent doesn't necessarily give you the right to make or sell or even use your own invention. You just get the right to keep *others* from making or using or selling it.

Peter: Huh. How come?

Michael: Well, let's say you develop a new chip design that doubles computer speed. You can patent your design, but that doesn't give you the right to make and sell an entire computer, or maybe not even the chip itself. A whole bunch of other people may hold patents on a whole bunch of the other components. So with your patent, you can go to Apple® and offer to license your invention to them, in return for royalties. Or you could sell your patent to Dell® and they might use it, or license it to other companies, or they might just sit on it to keep anybody else from using it until it expires. But that's another bedtime story. We need to get back to the three patents.

Amy: I'm still waiting for the suspense part.

Michael: We're getting there. See, for a long time people had a pretty clear idea about what kinds of things were patentable within those three patenting regimes. And people had a pretty clear idea about what kinds of things weren't patentable. For instance, pure ideas or thought processes weren't patentable. Languages weren't patentable. Business practices weren't patentable. Mathematic and scientific laws and equations and theories weren't patentable. Products of nature weren't patentable—except for those domesticated plants and the occasional highly purified substance. And then along came computers and the genetic revolution, and they totally upset the apple cart.

Peter: Oh, right—because I could patent my chip, but what if I'm a code writer? Am I allowed to patent my code? Or do I just get a copyright?

Michael: Precisely. Copyright would keep someone from reproducing the text of your software, but its value doesn't lie in the text itself. The program functions within the computer as a kind of process—and processes are patentable. So how do we treat software? And then, when the Internet came along there was a big fuss about the 'business practice' exclusion because people wanted to be able to patent new ways of shopping and paying bills online. So that's been an area of contention, too.

But returning to genetics... the watershed case here is *Diamond v. Chakrabarty*,[6] from the early 1980s.

This guy Chakrabarty worked in R&D at GE®, and he developed a new strain of bacteria to digest oil in oil spills. Long before him, scientists had discovered naturally occurring bacteria that digested certain fractions of oil, and the industry used combinations of these bacteria to help clear oil slicks. But it was hard to keep the proportions right—so you'd still be left with undigested oil. Chakrabarty knew that the capacity to digest the oil fractions rested in little symbiotic rings of DNA within the bacteria, called *plasmids*. Each strain of bacteria had its own strain of plasmid. So he took the plasmids from four strains of bacteria and combined them in a single host bacterium, to make a sort of super-bug that could digest four different fractions of oil. Pretty clever, right?

Peter: I'm impressed.

Michael: Me, too. Next, Chakrabarty and GE® applied for a utility patent. They asked for coverage of the bacterium itself, for the process of making it and keeping it stable, and for the method of using it on oil spills. The Patent Office granted the process and method claims, but they refused to patent the actual bacterium because they said living organisms couldn't be patented. GE® and Chakrabarty filed an appeal in court. That's where "Diamond" comes in—he was the head of the PTO, the Patent and Trademark Office, at the time. Eventually this case found its way to the Supreme Court, and they ruled in favor of Chakrabarty—about a decade after his initial patent application, by the way. The Supreme Court said it was irrelevant that a living organism was involved, because the invention produced something not previously found in nature.

Amy: Sounds reasonable to me.

Michael: Yeah—a lot of people thought so. But a lot of people were worried, too. Like, what if humans themselves could be patented? There was a pretty clear answer to that in the prohibition against slavery, but nobody really knew what the new boundaries were.

Another spectacular thing that happened around that time was PCR—polymerase chain reaction. Some people called it a "molecular Xerox® machine." It lets you take a small amount of DNA and make tons of copies. It's fast and cheap. Along with better ways to sequence DNA, it really speeded up genetic discovery. And that's when I think things started to go a little screwy in the PTO.

Amy: You're talking mid-eighties here, right? When the Human Genome Project got started?

Michael: Yep. A three billion–dollar project to figure out the genetic code of human beings. So lots of money, lots of scientists, lots of commercial opportunity. And in the early years, people were still figuring out the technology and it was a really big deal to identify and isolate a gene. So this entirely new class of applications started coming into the Patent Office, based on gene sequences from living organisms.

The PTO could have interpreted *Chakrabarty* narrowly, to allow patents only on recombinant products not found in nature—like a gene for human insulin embedded in a yeast that will churn out insulin. Instead, the PTO began allowing patents for the gene sequences themselves.

Amy: How could they, if those genes are products of nature?

Michael: Workarounds. The applications were careful to avoid claiming native DNA or raw sequence data. Instead, the claims were for "purified DNA molecules," or "intronless sequences," that sort of thing.[7]

Amy: "Intronless sequences?"

Michael: Yeah, I guess it's been awhile since our college biology course, hasn't it? Remember, genes are broken up into coding and noncoding regions. The parts that get translated into proteins are the "exons" and the parts that get taken out before translation are the "introns."

Peter: How on earth do you remember that?

Michael: I think of the **ex**ons as the parts that **ex**it to become protein, and the **in**trons as the parts that stay **in** the nucleus. I have no idea whether that's the real reason for the names. So anyway, an "intronless sequence" would be essentially the recipe for the protein, with no extraneous information.

Amy: So does this mean somebody who holds a patent on a gene owns the genes and proteins my own body makes?

Michael: Nobody ever tried to claim his or her patents went that far. After all, the money was in the commercial and scientific use of the discoveries, not in how the human body used its genes. So they argued that the molecules isolated and sequenced in their labs weren't the same ones found in nature.[8]

Joy: Okay, now you're saying "discoveries" instead of "inventions." Which is it?

Michael: Sorry. It's both. The actual language is "whoever invents or discovers any new and useful process, machine, manufacture, or composition of matter."[3] The intent was to exclude purely scientific discoveries but still allow people to patent new ways to harness those discoveries. If you discovered a new, naturally occurring mineral, you couldn't patent the mineral itself. But if you developed a method of extracting or producing or refining the mineral, you could patent that method. And if you developed a way to use the mineral, you could patent that use.

Joy: I can patent my new mineral as a component of glazes, but I can't patent the mineral itself, even though that would be a lot better for me. So why is there a different rule for genes?

Michael: Well, that's exactly the question people have been asking.

One argument is that the PTO had a history of allowing patents on highly purified versions of naturally occurring molecules. In the early 1900s a patent was upheld not only for the process of extracting adrenaline from cattle, but also for adrenaline itself, even though those cattle obviously made that adrenaline while they were alive.[9] I guess there's some question about whether the extracted molecule was truly identical to the original—but I'm not sure they could have figured that out at the time. Anyway, the adrenaline case stands for the principle that highly purified, naturally occurring substances may be patentable. But it was really rare until the gene patents started getting issued.

Peter: It seems to me there's a big difference between patenting extracted adrenaline and patenting the gene for adrenaline. I mean, the genetic sequence is fundamental—it almost feels like copyrighting the alphabet.

Michael: . . . or is it like patenting a computer program? Both codes initiate a process that produces a product.

Peter: Well, program code is written by people. Genes aren't.

Michael: Good point. In fact, I don't think anybody's quarrelling about whether you can patent artificially created genes. Or their products. It's the stranglehold on naturally occurring sequences that's under scrutiny.

Amy: Wait—if people have patents on "purified sequences," how come that gives them a stranglehold on the natural genes?

Michael: The patent holders said anytime you used their claimed gene sequences in the lab, you were reproducing their purified sequences and infringing upon their patents[10,11] They were careful to cover all the permutations. So, they'd claim the sequence itself, along with the reverse sequence, the RNA sequence, the amino acid sequence, and any probes to the sequence . . . so they really had you boxed in, not only if you were a diagnostic lab but also if you were a primary research lab.

Patients looking for diagnostic tests sometimes ended up having to be tested more than once because company Q claimed a handful of mutations, and company R claimed some others. Neither could report on the other's mutations—so if Q found one of R's mutations, all it could say was that the person should be tested by R.[2] You remember reading in the paper that Myriad held patents to the breast cancer genes, BRCA1 and BRCA2?

Joy: Yeah.

Michael: At least it was one-stop shopping. Everybody sent their samples to Myriad—which meant Myriad was the first to "discover" mutations that cause cancer—and for awhile they filed new patent applications on those mutations as they found them. So even though their original patents would run out eventually, they'd still have fresh patents on newly discovered mutations, and any other diagnostic lab that found those mutations and reported them would be infringing until those newer patents ran out.

Joy: But Myriad was sued, right?

Michael: Right. A bunch of people got together and sued Myriad and the PTO.[3] In the lower courts they argued that the BRCA gene sequence patents were invalid because the sequences were products of nature. And they argued that a bunch of the method patents were invalid, too. Myriad was the perfect target because it had pretty much a total monopoly on testing for those two genes.[14] According to the petitioners, if you wanted a second opinion you couldn't get one; Myriad didn't always take Medicaid, so if you were covered by Medicaid you couldn't get tested at all;[15] and it enforced its patents against breast cancer researchers as well as diagnostic labs—although it said it was willing to sequence the genes for researchers at cost.[15] So Myriad had some PR problems to begin with—and people assumed it had deep pockets so it could afford to put up a fight.

I have to say, because of its monopoly, Myriad has been able to build a really impressive database linking gene mutations with information about how those mutations played out in real life—which probably wouldn't have happened if the testing had been spread over a bunch of labs. And they sent updates to patients they'd tested in the past if they found something new about the patients' mutations. So that part of their business was really admirable. Myriad also figured out a long time ago that it wasn't in the company's best interest to keep publishing all the mutations it found—so it stopped filing patent applications and started keeping that accumulated information private. But in those original patent applications, the drafters really pushed the margins on their claims. So they were ripe for challenge.

Peter: How so?

Michael: Well, not only did they claim all of the normal sequences and the mutations they found early on, but they claimed *any variation* from the normal gene sequence, whether or not Myriad discovered it.[6] How the heck did that get past the PTO?

And their method patents described stuff that seems really obvious—like comparing the gene sequence of a tumor sample to the gene sequence of a nontumor sample, and intuiting that any differences you find are new mutations that caused the tumor.[17] Or using cell cultures with various BRCA mutations to test the efficacy of cancer drugs against those mutations.[18] People had been performing those operations for years—so why was it patentable just because you're using BRCA genes? Trouble was, once the PTO agreed to a claim like that for one applicant it was harder to back down the next time.

In fact, method claims very similar to Myriad's were overturned a little while ago in a court case involving the Mayo Clinic's® labs.[19] Mayo® developed a new way to measure the levels of a drug byproduct in peoples' blood samples, and they got sued by a lab called Prometheus® that held patents to an older test. Prometheus® held patents not only to its original test kits, but also to the process of comparing the patient's blood level to the optimal level and then adjusting the drug dose accordingly. So Prometheus® argued that no matter how you measured the blood level, it held the rights to the comparison and adjustment. The Supreme Court sided with Mayo® and said those claims weren't valid. They said "laws of nature, natural phenomena and abstract ideas" couldn't be turned into patentable subject matter simply by reciting them or instructing people to apply them.

Joy: It's like saying, "hold your glass under the tap, turn it on, and use gravity to fill the glass with water."

Michael: Exactly. To be fair, back when those early genes were discovered and sequenced it was really dazzling. But after awhile it got to be grunt work. Mostly automated. Even apart from the products of nature argument, I think years ago the PTO should have put the brakes on gene patents because of obviousness. There's no inventive concept anymore to the isolation and sequencing. And I'm suspicious of a lot of the method patents for the same reason.

Amy: So, what happened with the Myriad lawsuit?

Michael: Well, the Supreme Court issued a unanimous decision saying naturally occurring gene sequences can't be patented[20] But it said cDNA is patent-eligible because it isn't found in nature.[20,21] cDNA is "complementary DNA"—you get it by retranslating the RNA coding sequence back into its DNA counterpart. It's essentially like intronless DNA.

The Court didn't actually consider any of the method patents in *Myriad*—it just agreed to review the patent eligibility of naturally occurring sequences. So Myriad will probably be challenged next on its method patents. And the Court kind of hinted that the PTO should take a harder look at its novelty and non-obviousness criteria.[22]

Joy: Help me out again—sometimes you say "patentability" and sometimes you say "patent eligibility"—wouldn't they be the same things?

Michael: Not quite. Patent *eligibility* is the first hurdle. Eligibility asks whether this is a product or a process that could be patented if it meets the other criteria. *Patentability* is the second set of hurdles. Patentability hinges on novelty, utility, obviousness—and a whole bunch of other procedural stuff. So by saying native DNA is not *patent eligible*, the Supreme Court Justices said you can't even reach the questions of novelty, utility and non-obviousness with naturally occurring DNA. But a month earlier, the Court had published another unanimous opinion essentially upholding a patent on artificially-constructed DNA.[23]

Amy: Oh, yeah—we haven't talked about Monsanto yet.

Michael: Right. This kind of brings us back to *Chakrabarty*.

Amy: I think I'm seeing the link.

Michael: I bet you are. So, imagine you're Monsanto. You've done some actual genetic engineering to develop your Roundup®-ready corn—you've inserted a gene that previously didn't exist in nature, to create a plant that previously didn't exist in nature. This plant is resistant to an herbicide that previously didn't exist in nature. The only commercial value in your invention is going to be through seed-propagated plants—so a plant patent is useless. But *Chakrabarty* has opened the door for you to get a utility patent for your plant, so you patent the method of making Roundup® resistant plants, and you also patent the corn or the beans or whatever you're selling—which is really revolutionary, because it totally sidesteps the plant patent limitations. But now you run into another problem.

Remember our example of a new way to make shoes? Let's say I've invented a totally new machine that makes formed plastic shoes, where you can dial in all the shape specifications and mold just the shoe you want. I build that machine and I sell it to a shoemaker.

Joy: I want one.

Michael: Done. Now, when you buy my machine you don't have the right to make and sell copies of the machine. But if you decide to sell my machine to your neighbor you can, and you won't owe me anything. My patent rights in that particular machine are "exhausted" after the first sale. If I want a say in the future possession of my machine, then instead of selling it I have to lease it to you.

More importantly, you have the right to make and sell the shoes you produce using my machine without owing me anything. In fact, that's the only reason you'd buy the equipment in the first place. You own those shoes outright, you can sell them to whomever you choose, and your customers can sell them to whomever they choose. In the past there's always been a bright line between the manufacturing *process* and the *product* of manufacture, because there's always been a clear distinction between the machine and the product of the machine.

Amy: But not with Monsanto's seeds.

Michael: But not with Monsanto's seeds. With Monsanto's seeds, the product and the machine are, essentially, one and the same. If I buy a bushel of seed corn and grow it, I'll get maybe 500 bushels of corn from my crop. I could save a bushel and sell 499, and plant that saved bushel the next year for another 500-bushel yield. And I'd never have to darken Monsanto's door again. So Monsanto has been aggressive about enforcing its patent against farmers who try to replant or sell to someone else for planting. It's almost like the farmers don't actually own the seed—they just get a license to grow a year's crop and use or sell it for nonseed purposes.

Joy: So why is this so different from before? I don't remember seed suppliers giving farmers a hard time about replanting when I was a kid.

Michael: Well, I was kind of lying about that second 500-bushel yield, wasn't I? I think then and now most seeds are hybrids made the old fashioned way, by crossing two parent strains. So the first daughter strain is going to be really uniform and have certain desired characteristics. But after that first generation, those seeds will have random recombinations and the crop won't have the same value. You could "replant," sure—especially if you're growing for silage—but you really wouldn't be competing with the seed companies. Your neighbors probably wouldn't be interested in buying your random corn for their own crops.

But with these new genetically engineered strains, the inserted genes are going to persist through multiple generations, for good or ill, regardless of the genetic background of the rest of the seed. And that's how Vernon Bowman ended up in court.

Joy: He's the farmer who got sued by Monsanto?

Michael: He's one of hundreds who have run afoul of Monsanto. He's just more stubborn than the rest. Bowman was in the habit of buying Monsanto's soybeans for his first crop of the year, and selling his harvest to the grain elevator. But for the second crop, which was more iffy from a weather standpoint, instead of buying from Monsanto he planted beans he purchased from the elevator. That way he could claim he didn't "replant" the beans he grew under his original contract with Monsanto. But he knew that most of the beans in that elevator were probably Roundup® resistant beans. And then—as if to thumb his nose at Monsanto—he treated his second crop with Roundup®, so of course he killed any beans that didn't have the Roundup®-resistant gene. He did this for years.[23]

Joy: I assume the Supreme Court wasn't impressed.

Michael: You're right. The Supreme Court Justices agreed with Monsanto that planting those beans constituted a violation of the patent, because Bowman essentially was making copies of Monsanto's machine. It also reaffirmed the *Chakrabarty* principle that genetically engineered organisms are patent eligible, and essentially gave Monsanto the green light to keep making and patenting resistant crops.[23]

Amy: But won't that resistant gene get into the wild eventually? Will Monsanto claim every plant in the world that contains its gene?

Michael: There's a sad idea. You're right—if history is any guide, that gene will eventually cross over into other plants—which will be a shame, because I like Roundup® and at some point it won't work anymore. But by then, Monsanto's patent on the resistant gene will have expired. No doubt they're working on some new herbicide and gene combo for their next generation of products. Who knows? Maybe herbicide companies are hoping Roundup® resistance becomes widespread, to clear the way for other compounds.

Joy: And in the meantime, organic farmers are terrified that the gene will get into their crops and ruin their markets. Can they sue Monsanto for contaminating their crops?

Michael: Probably... I'm not sure anyone has tried. They might claim reckless endangerment of property or something. It wouldn't be easy.

Joy: So as it stands, we have patent protection for Frankenfoods but not for normal or abnormal sequences in humans. How will that affect companies working on human diseases?

Peter: Myriad will have some competition, that's for sure.

Michael: I heard other labs started offering BRCA testing within hours after the opinion was published, but I'm guessing Myriad will do just fine. That huge database will give it a powerful edge. And they could still try to enforce their method patents, but it seems like a losing battle to me. I do think this case will make testing cheaper and more readily available. And it'll make it a lot easier to put together comprehensive tests for thousands of different conditions—where with private ownership of genes it would be a nightmare.

Amy: And researchers are happy, I bet.

Michael: I think basic science labs are breathing sighs of relief, but I'm not sure whether it will help or hurt commercial development. Startups really push their ability to acquire patent protection when they look for investors. Still, artificially engineered products should be eligible for protection under these new rulings. It just won't feel like such a sure thing.

Amy: Well, here's hoping somebody is working on early-onset Alzheimer.

Peter: I'll drink to that.

REFERENCES

1. 35 U.S. Code § 171—Patents for designs

   Whoever invents any new, original and ornamental design for an article of manufacture may obtain a patent therefor, subject to the conditions and requirements of this title.

2. 35 U.S. Code § 161—Patents for plants

   Whoever invents or discovers and asexually reproduces any distinct and new variety of plant, including cultivated sports, mutants, hybrids, and newly found seedlings, other than a tuber propagated plant or a plant found in an uncultivated state, may obtain a patent therefor, subject to the conditions and requirements of this title.

3. 35 U.S. Code § 101—Inventions patentable

   Whoever invents or discovers any new and useful process, machine, manufacture, or composition of matter, or any new and useful improvement thereof, may obtain a patent therefor, subject to the conditions and requirements of this title.

4. 35 U.S. Code § 102 (a)—Novelty; prior art

   A person shall be entitled to a patent unless—
   (1) the claimed invention was patented, described in a printed publication, or in public use, on sale, or otherwise available to the public before the effective filing date of the claimed invention;
   [other provisions and exceptions follow in this section]

5. 35 U.S. Code § 103—Conditions for patentability; non-obvious subject matter

   A patent for a claimed invention may not be obtained, notwithstanding that the claimed invention is not identically disclosed as set forth in section 102, if the differences between the claimed invention and the prior art are such that the claimed invention as a whole would have been obvious before the effective filing date of the claimed invention to a person having ordinary skill in the art to which the claimed invention pertains. Patentability shall not be negated by the manner in which the invention was made.

6. *Diamond v. Chakrabarty*, 447 U.S. 303 (1980)

7. Claims from US Patent 6,984,487 Cystic Fibrosis Gene (2006)

1. A purified DNA molecule, comprising a cystic fibrosis transmembrane conductance regulator (CFTR) DNA sequence selected from the group consisting of:

(a) a DNA sequence encoding a normal CFTR protein having the amino acid sequence depicted in FIG. 1;

(b) a DNA sequence which hybridizes under stringent conditions to at least 16 contiguous nucleotides of the DNA sequence depicted in FIG. 1; and

(c) a DNA sequence complementary to the DNA sequence of (a) or (b), wherein said DNA sequence of (a), (b) or (c), when present as part of a coding sequence of a normal CFTR gene, is expressed in human epithelial cells as a normal CFTR protein which is not characterized as having cystic fibrosis associated activity.

2. A purified normal CFTR RNA molecule, comprising an RNA sequence having the DNA sequence recited in claim 1, wherein, in said RNA sequence, each thymidylate in said DNA sequence is replaced with a uridine.

3. A purified DNA molecule according to claim 1, wherein said purified DNA molecule is cDNA.

[...]

Claims from US Patent 5,654,170 Polycystic Kidney Disease Gene (1997)

1. Isolated nucleic acid comprising the sequence set forth in SEQ ID NO:1 or its complement.

2. Isolated nucleic acid according to claim 1 wherein said nucleic acid is RNA.

3. Isolated nucleic acid comprising an intronless sequence derived from the sequence of claim 1 wherein said nucleic acid is cDNA.

4. A recombinant cloning vector comprising the nucleic acid of claim 3.

5. The vector of claim 4 further comprising a transcriptional regulatory element operably linked to said nucleic acid, said element having the ability to direct the expression of

genes of prokaryotic or eukaryotic cells and their viruses or combinations thereof.

6. A cell comprising the vector of claim 5.

7. A method for producing a recombinant protein, said method comprising:

(a) culturing the cell of claim 6 in a medium and under conditions suitable for expression of said protein, and

(b) isolating said expressed protein.

8. An isolated nucleic acid comprising the sequence set forth in SEQ ID NO:2.

9. An isolated nucleic acid comprising 5'AGGACCTGT CCAGGCATC-3' SEQ ID NO:8.

8. Brief for Respondents, *Myriad*

[1.] [. . .] No one would doubt the patent-eligibility of a newly-created chemical composition that, when applied in a laboratory to a person's blood or tissue sample, could detect a mutation genetically predisposing her to a risk of breast or ovarian cancer, thereby allowing her to take proactive measures to prolong her life even before cancer actually strikes. That is what Myriad's patented molecules are—and they were never available to the world until Myriad's scientists applied their inventive faculties to a previously undistinguished mass of genetic matter in order to identify, define, and create the isolated DNA molecules.

[2.] It has long been established that specific isolated molecules of deoxyribonucleic acid ("DNA") are patent-eligible. "Isolated" means that a human being has defined the molecule and separated it from the complex of genetic material that accompanies it in the body, or (as with complementary DNA, or cDNA) synthetically created the molecule in a laboratory. Such molecules may include recombinant, cloned, or synthesized DNA isolates. This human design and action transforms the molecule's physical structure and alters its chemistry.

[. . .]

As the patents describe, the specific isolated BRCA1 and BRCA2 molecules, once defined, were either separated from surrounding genomic and cellular matter at precise locations chosen by the Myriad inventors, or assembled in a laboratory (in the case of cDNA). Their human inventive choices defined the particular isolated molecules, free from genetic and other surrounding material, to enable their utility outside the body in ways that naturally-occurring DNA in the body lacks. To function within the body, a gene cannot be isolated, but must be physically bound to other genes, nucleic acids, and proteins within the chromosome.

No. 12-398 Supreme Court of the United States, *Association of Molecular Pathology et al. v. Myriad Genetics, Inc., et al.*, Brief for Respondents, pages 1, 6-7. Available at: http://www.americanbar.org/content/dam/aba/publications/supreme_court_preview/briefs-v2/12-398_resp.authcheckdam.pdf. Accessed July 5, 2013.

9. *Parke-Davis & Co. v. H.K. Mulford Co.*, 189 F. 95 (1911)
10. Brief for Petitioners, *Myriad*

Myriad defends its claims on the grounds that a gene becomes a human invention when removed from the human body ("isolated"). Under this rationale, a kidney "isolated" from the body would be patentable, gold "isolated" from a stream would be patentable, and leaves "isolated" from trees would be patentable. This defense defies common sense and elevates the draftsman's art over the long-standing prohibition on patenting of products and laws of nature.

Because it is not possible to study or use the genes unless they are isolated, the claims have significant implications. The claims preempt any use of the genes for any purpose. [...] Although Myriad has not exercised its authority to stop all research, Myriad's claims have had a proven chilling effect on research, as laboratories are dissuaded from pursuing scientific work that requires using the patented genes.

Even more disturbingly, because the claims reach all possible uses of the claimed genes, Myriad is authorized to block avenues of scientific inquiry. Myriad can prevent researchers from determining if mutations on the genes correlate with increased risk of other diseases. It can prevent researchers from determining whether the genes could be used in therapy, and if they could, Myriad can prevent that use or lay claim to it. Myriad can stop the development of new types of clinical testing of the genes that take advantage of recent scientific insights. If it were determined that the genes could be used for purposes not now known, such as a substitute for silicon chips in computers (a use currently being explored by companies), Myriad can prevent that use. Myriad can even prevent scientists from looking at their own genes.

No. 12-398 Supreme Court of the United States, *Association of Molecular Pathology et al v. Myriad Genetics, Inc., et al*, Brief for Petitioners, pages 2–3. Available at: http://www.americanbar.org/content/dam/aba/publications/supreme_court_preview/briefs-v2/12-398_pet.authcheckdam.pdf. Accessed July 5, 2013.

11. Supreme Court Opinion, *Myriad*

    Myriad's patents would, if valid, give it the exclusive right to isolate an individual's BRCA1 and BRCA2 genes (or any strand of 15 or more nucleotides within the genes) by breaking the covalent bonds that connect the DNA to the rest of the individual's genome. The patents would also give Myriad the exclusive right to synthetically create BRCA cDNA. In Myriad's view, manipulating BRCA DNA in either of these fashions triggers its "right to exclude others from making" its patented composition of matter under the Patent Act.

    Association for Molecular Pathology v. Myriad Genetics, Inc., et al., 569 U.S.___(2013) slip opinion, at 6.

12. Secretary's Advisory Committee on Genetics, Health and Society: Gene Patents and Licensing Practices and Patient Access to Genetic Tests *(Public Consultation Report March 2009)*. See especially discussion of genes associated with hearing loss. Accessed March 1, 2013 at: http://oba.od.nih.gov/SACGHS/sacghs_documents.html#GHSDOC_011.

13. *Association for Molecular Pathology, et al. v. Myriad Genetics, Inc., et al.*, 569 U.S. ___ (2013).

Lower court decisions:

Association for Molecular Pathology v. United States Patent and Trademark Office, 689 F.3d 1303 (Fed. Cir. 2012)

Association for Molecular Pathology v. United States Patent and Trademark Office, 653 F.3d 1329 (Fed. Cir. 2011)

Association for Molecular Pathology v. United States Patent and Trademark Office, 702 F.Supp.2d 181 (S.D.N.Y. 2010)

14. Interestingly, a study by ethicists at Duke University compared the per-amplicon cost of BRCA1–2 testing with those of tests for unpatented genes, offered by multiple labs. The study found Myriad's BRCA1–2 prices fell within the range of the per-amplicon prices for the tests offered by other vendors. **Secretary's Advisory Committee on Genetics, Health and Society: Gene Patents and Licensing Practices and Patient Access to Genetic Tests** *(Public Consultation Report March 2009). See especially Appendix A: Compendium of Case Studies Prepared for SACGHS by the Duke University Center for Genome Ethics, Law & Policy by Cook-Deegan et al.* Accessed March 1, 2013 at http://oba.od.nih.gov/SACGHS/sacghs_documents.html#GHSDOC_011.

15. Complaint filed at initiation of *Association for Molecular Pathology v. United States Patent and Trademark Office*, 702 F.Supp.2d 191, (2010) Southern District of New York. Accessed March 1, 2013 at http://www.aclu.org/free-speech/brca-complaint.

16. U.S. Patent Number 5,837,492 Chromosome 13-linked Breast Cancer Susceptibility Gene (1998) claim #6 reads:

    6. An isolated DNA molecule coding for a mutated form of the BRCA2 polypeptide set forth in SEQ ID NO:2, wherein said mutated form of the BRCA2 polypeptide is *associated with susceptibility* to cancer. *(emphasis added)*

17. U.S. Patent Number 6,033,857 Chromosome 13-linked Breast Cancer Susceptibility Gene (2000) claim #1 reads:

    1. A method for identifying a mutant BRCA2 nucleotide sequence in a suspected mutant BRCA2 allele which comprises

comparing the nucleotide sequence of the suspected mutant BRCA2 allele with the wild-type BRCA2 nucleotide sequence, wherein *a difference between the suspected mutant and the wild-type sequences identifies a mutant* BRCA2 nucleotide sequence. *(emphasis added)*

U.S. Patent Number 5,710,001 17q-linked Breast and Ovarian Cancer Susceptibility Gene (1998) claim #1 reads:

1. A method for screening a tumor sample from a human subject for a somatic alteration in a BRCA1 gene in said tumor which comprises comparing a first sequence selected from the group consisting of a BRCA1 gene from said tumor sample, BRCA1 RNA from said tumor sample and BRCA1 cDNA made from mRNA from said tumor sample with a second sequence selected from the group consisting of BRCA1 gene from a nontumor sample of said subject, BRCA1 RNA from said nontumor sample and BRCA1 cDNA made from mRNA from said nontumor sample, wherein *a difference in the sequence of the BRCA1 gene, BRCA1 RNA or BRCA1 cDNA from said tumor sample from the sequence of the BRCA1 gene, BRCA1 RNA or BRCA1 cDNA from said nontumor sample indicates a somatic alteration in the BRCA1 gene in said tumor sample. (emphasis added)*

18. U.S. Patent Number 5,747,282 17q-linked Breast and Ovarian Cancer Susceptibility Gene (1998) claim # 20 reads:

20. A method for screening potential cancer therapeutics which comprises: *growing a transformed eukaryotic host cell containing an altered BRCA1 gene causing cancer in the presence of a compound suspected of being a cancer therapeutic*, growing said transformed eukaryotic host cell in the absence of said compound, determining the rate of growth of said host cell in the presence of said compound and the rate of growth of said host cell in the absence of said compound and *comparing the growth rate* of said host cells, wherein a slower rate of growth of said host cell in the presence of said compound is indicative of a cancer therapeutic. (*emphasis added*)

19. Supreme Court Opinion, *Mayo*

> The Court has long held that [section 101] contains an important implicit exception. "[L]aws of nature, natural phenomena, and abstract ideas" are not patentable. *Diamond v. Diehr,* 450 U.S. 175, 185 (1981)...
>
> *Mayo Collaborative Services v. Prometheus Labs., Inc.*, 132 S. Ct. 1289, at 1293

> [Prior cases] insist that a process that focuses upon the use of a natural law also contain other elements or a combination of elements, sometimes referred to as an "inventive concept," sufficient to ensure that the patent in practice amounts to significantly more than a patent upon the natural law itself. [*Parker v. Flook,* 437 U.S. 584].
>
> *Mayo Collaborative Services v. Prometheus Labs., Inc.*, 132 S. Ct. 1289, at 1294

> We find that the process claims at issue here do not satisfy these conditions. In particular, the steps in the claimed processes (apart from the natural laws themselves) involve well-understood, routine, conventional activity previously engaged in by researchers in the field. At the same time, upholding the patents would risk disproportionately tying up the use of the underlying natural laws, inhibiting their use in the making of further discoveries.
>
> *Mayo Collaborative Services v. Prometheus Labs., Inc.*, 132 S. Ct. 1289, at 1294

20. Supreme Court Opinion, *Myriad*

> For the reasons that follow, we hold that a naturally occurring DNA segment is a product of nature and not patent eligible merely because it has been isolated, but that cDNA is patent eligible because it is not naturally occurring.
>
> *Association for Molecular Pathology, et al. v. Myriad Genetics, Inc., et al.*, 569 U.S. ___ (2013) slip opinion, at 1.

> It is undisputed that Myriad did not create or alter any of the genetic information encoded in the BRCA1 and BRCA2 genes.

The location and order of the nucleotides existed in nature before Myriad found them. Nor did Myriad create or alter the genetic structure of DNA. Instead, Myriad's principal contribution was uncovering the precise location and genetic sequence of the BRCA1 and BRCA2 genes within chromosomes 17 and 13. The question is whether this renders the genes patentable. [. . .] The Chakrabarty bacterium was new "with markedly different characteristics from any found in nature," 447 U.S. 303, at 310, due to the additional plasmids and resultant "capacity for degrading oil." Id., at 305, n.1. In this case, by contrast, Myriad did not create anything. To be sure, it found an important and useful gene, but separating that gene from its surrounding genetic material is not an act of invention.

Association for Molecular Pathology, et al. v. Myriad Genetics, Inc., et al., 569 U.S. ___ (2013) slip opinion, at 11–12

Nor are Myriad's claims saved by the fact that isolating DNA from the human genome severs chemical bonds and thereby creates a nonnaturally occurring molecule. Myriad's claims are simply not expressed in terms of chemical composition, nor do they rely in any way on the chemical changes that result from the isolation of a particular section of DNA. Instead, the claims understandably focus on the genetic information encoded in the BRCA1 and BRCA2 genes. If the patents depended upon the creation of a unique molecule, then a would-be infringer could arguably avoid at least Myriad's patent claims on entire genes (such as claims 1 and 2 of the '282 patent) by isolating a DNA sequence and one additional nucleotide pair. Such a molecule would not be chemically identical to the molecule "invented" by Myriad. But Myriad obviously would resist that outcome because its claim is concerned primarily with the information contained in the genetic sequence, not with the specific chemical composition of a particular molecule.

Finally, Myriad argues that the PTO's past practice of awarding gene patents is entitled to deference, citing *J.E.M. Ag Supply, Inc. v. Pioneer HiBred Int'l, Inc*, 534 U.S. 124 (2001). We disagree.

Association for Molecular Pathology, et al. v. Myriad Genetics, Inc., et al., 569 U.S. ___ (2013) slip opinion, at 14–15

21. Supreme Court Opinion, *Myriad*

cDNA does not present the same obstacles to patentability as naturally occurring, isolated DNA segments. As already explained, creation of a cDNA sequence from mRNA results in an exons-only molecule that is not naturally occurring. Petitioners concede that cDNA differs from natural DNA in that "the non-coding regions have been removed." They nevertheless argue that cDNA is not patent eligible because "[t]he nucleotide sequence of cDNA is dictated by nature not by the lab technician." That may be so, but the lab technician unquestionably creates something new when cDNA is made. cDNA retains the naturally occurring exons of DNA, but it is distinct from the DNA from which it was derived. As a result, cDNA is not a "product of nature" and is patent eligible under §101, except insofar as very short series of DNA may have no intervening introns to remove when creating cDNA. In that situation, a short strand of cDNA may be indistinguishable from natural DNA.

Association for Molecular Pathology, et al. v. Myriad Genetics, Inc., et al., 569 U.S. ___(2013) slip opinion, at 16–17.

22. Supreme Court Opinion, *Myriad*

DNA's informational sequences and the processes that create mRNA, amino acids, and proteins occur naturally within cells. Scientists can, however, extract DNA from cells using *well known* laboratory methods. These methods allow scientists to isolate specific segments of DNA—for instance, a particular gene or part of a gene—which can then be further studied, manipulated, or used. It is also possible to create DNA synthetically through processes similarly *well known* in the field of genetics. *(emphasis added)*

Association for Molecular Pathology, et al. v. Myriad Genetics, Inc., et al., 569 U.S. ___(2013) slip opinion, at 3.

It is important to note what is *not* implicated by this decision. First, there are no method claims before this Court. Had Myriad created an innovative method of manipulating genes while searching for the BRCA1 and BRCA2 genes, it could possibly have sought a method patent. But the processes used by Myriad to isolate DNA... at the time of Myriad's patents "*were well understood, widely used, and fairly uniform* insofar as any scientist engaged in the search for a gene would likely have utilized a similar approach," 702 F. Supp. 2d, at 202–203, and are not at issue in this case. *(emphasis added in last sentence)*

Association for Molecular Pathology, et al. v. Myriad Genetics, Inc., et al., 569 U.S. ___(2013) slip opinion, at 17. See also footnote 19.

23. Supreme Court Opinion, *Monsanto*

Under the doctrine of patent exhaustion, the authorized sale of a patented article gives the purchaser, or any subsequent owner, a right to use or resell that article. Such a sale, however, does not allow the purchaser to make new copies of the patented invention. The question in this case is whether a farmer who buys patented seeds may reproduce them through planting and harvesting without the patent holder's permission. We hold that he may not.

Bowman v. Monsanto Co., 569 U.S. ___ (2013) slip opinion, at 1.

8

Ethical Issues in Genetic and Genomic Research

DAWN C. ALLAIN AND KELLY E. ORMOND

In this chapter we will review principles of human subjects research as they apply to genetic and genomic research. This will include a review of international and US-based guidelines and regulatory bodies. We will then discuss cross-cutting ethical issues, using research examples including privacy and data-sharing issues, return of results, commercialization issues and investigator conflicts of interest, multiple use of samples, withdrawal from research, and informed consent.

The types of human subject research in medicine vary, but most have similar goals. Researchers and medical professionals want to delineate the underlying cause and natural history of disease, develop diagnostic technologies, implement targeted therapeutic interventions, and improve patient outcomes. However, while performing the research necessary to gather this knowledge researchers must balance the benefits and risks to the human subjects involved. In addition, the human subject's rights, interests, and overall health status must be taken into account. Each country has different regulatory approaches to human subjects research. In the United States (which we will focus on), the use of human subjects in research is regulated by the federal government; international regulations also exist.

Human subjects research is defined by the Federal Policy for the Protection of Human Subject Research (typically called the

"Common Rule" or 45CFR46) as research involving "a living individual about whom an investigator...conducting research obtains (1) data through intervention or interaction with the individual or (2) identifiable private information." In order to require oversight (most frequently by an institutional review board (IRB), a protocol must involve both "research" and "human subjects." In this chapter we provide an overview of guidelines surrounding human subjects research, historical and current examples of genetic research, and a discussion of some key ethical issues that arise in ethically performing such research.

Guidelines for Human Subject Research

International Guidelines

The Nuremberg Code (Box 8.1), written by judges and developed on the advice of medical experts who participated in the Nuremberg Trials, arose out of the Nuremberg Trials of 1947. This code, illustrated in Table 1, delineates 10 principles that were based on the premise that medical experimentation on human subjects must satisfy moral, ethical, and legal concepts.[1,2] It is clear from the first principle that informed consent from the subject is a required and valued criterion for performing research. In addition, many of the principles attend to the safety of the subject, the application of risk versus benefit ratios, and the idea that the research itself should be vetted for ethical acceptability. The obligations and responsibilities of both the subject and the investigator are also addressed by the Nuremberg Code. It is important to note that there is evidence to suggest that the Nuremberg Code itself was based on earlier published works.[2,3] However, it is the Nuremberg Code that has functioned as the basis for the responsible practice of medical research and is considered one of the landmark documents dealing with human subject research. Although it is accepted as an international guideline, one of the major problems with the Nuremberg code is that there is no way to enforce adherence to its principles because it is a recommendation, not an international law.[3] In addition, the Nuremberg Code has never been revised or updated over the years, so the principles still stand as first published in 1947. As such, other international and national guidelines/laws discussed in this chapter have been developed in subsequent years in order to guide human subject research.

The Declaration of Helsinki, the product of another international effort, was originally drafted by the World Medical Association in 1964. It was developed to clarify the principles put forth in the Nuremberg Code and to define the process of performing responsible human subjects research.[4] The Declaration of Helsinki was designed specifically to ensure the individual rights and safety of human subjects who participate in medical research. In addition it is targeted principally to physicians, although the document's preamble states that all individuals who participate in human subject research should adopt the principles within the document. Unlike the Nuremberg Code the Declaration of Helsinki has undergone seven revisions since its initial publication, with the most recent revision published in 2013.[5] The most recently revised document addresses human subject medical research as well as research on identifiable human material and data. It provides ethical and professional guidance for human subject research under the following subsections: general principles of medical research; risks, burdens and benefits; vulnerable groups and individuals; scientific requirements and research protocols; research ethics committees; privacy and confidentiality; use of placebo; post-trial provisions; research registration and publication and dissemination of results; and unproven interventions in clinical practice. Like the Nuremberg Code, the Declaration of Helsinki addresses issues of informed consent, safety, ethics, research design, subject withdrawal from research, minimization of risk, and maximization of benefits. The Declaration of Helsinki also specifically addresses the special consideration and protection of vulnerable research populations, regulatory and legal oversight, privacy of subjects, confidentiality of the subject's personal information, the concept of placebo-controlled trials, and the importance of public dissemination of negative, positive, and inconclusive research results. While the Declaration of Helsinki is a noted and well-respected internationally derived set of ethical principles it, like the Nuremberg Code, is unenforceable through international laws. However, although unenforceable on its own, the principles within the document have been used to develop national and international regulatory and legislative policies and have been codified in many of these policies and laws.

The World Medical Association adopted the Declaration on Ethical Considerations regarding Health Databases in 2002.[6] This document warrants being mentioned, as its principles were incorporated into the Declaration of Helsinki. Essentially the Declaration on Ethical Considerations regarding Health Databases addresses the right to privacy and confidentiality of an individual patient's personal health information (PHI), particularly data stored in databases. Thus when applying these guidelines to research, investigators must ensure that data was obtained with appropriate informed consent, that consent must be documented, subjects have a right to decline the storage of data for research purposes or request that it no longer be used/stored, and data can only be used for which authorization was obtained. In addition, databases must have safeguards in place to ensure that no inappropriate or unauthorized use of or access to the data occurs, and if data is used for secondary purposes it should be de-identified.

In addition, some international organizations have specifically addressed genetic research and genetic data.[7–10] For example, Article 5 of the United Nations Educational, Scientific and Cultural Organization (UNESCO) Universal Declaration on the Human Genome and Human Rights specifically addresses genetic research, stating that research on a person's genome shall only be undertaken after rigorous and prior assessment of the potential risks and benefits, uncoerced informed consent has been obtained, protocols have been reviewed in accordance with relevant national and international research standards/guidelines, and when an individual does not have the ability to consent, the research is being done only for the individual's direct health benefit.[9] UNESCO also developed a statement addressing human genetic data. Much like the 2002 WMA policy regarding Health Databases, UNESCO's Declaration on Human Genetic Data addresses concerns of access, privacy, and informed consent. However, UNESCO's declaration specifically addresses the special status of human genetic data—stating that it can be predictive of genetic disease, impact multiple generations, may at the time of collection may contain information of which the significance is not as yet known, and may have cultural significance.[9] Even the Organization for Economic Cooperation and Development (OECD), an international organization representing 34 countries whose mission is to promote policies to improve economic and social well-being of individuals throughout the world, developed guidelines for the development, oversight, implementation, access, use, and destruction of human biorepositories and genetic research databases.[7]

US Governmental Guidelines and Regulatory Bodies

In the United States, a number of documented and publicized abuses involving human subject research led the Congress to pass the 1974 National Research Act. This act established the creation of the National Commission for the Protection of Human Subjects of Biomedical and Behavioral Research within the Department of Health, Education, and Welfare. The charge of this committee was to establish distinctions between the boundaries required in human subject research versus standard of care or the routine practice of medicine.[11] This mandate led to the development of the well-known Belmont Report published in 1979 (described in chapter 1).[12] Essentially, the Belmont Report is a summary of the difference between biomedical research and medical practice and the identification of three ethical principles relevant to human subject research. It provides guidelines for how to resolve the ethical dilemmas that researchers may encounter while performing human subject research. Despite the international guidelines previously published, the Belmont Report is often cited as the sentinel document that set forth the three primary principles for ethical conduct of research: beneficence, justice, and respect for persons.[4,12–14] In the context of research these principles would be defined as follows: maximizing of benefits and reducing harm/minimizing risks of research on the subject (beneficence); ensuring autonomous decision making, also referred to as *informed consent* and *protection of vulnerable populations* (respect for persons); acknowledging the risks and benefits of the research; and disseminating the results of research findings (justice).[13,14]

The US Department of Health and Human Services (HHS) revised and expanded human subject regulation, establishing regulation referred to as 45CFR46. 45CFR46 policies require that any research funded by a federal department or agency must comply with the sections within the policy and must be reviewed and approved by an institutional review board (IRB) that adheres to the policy requirements. This regulation includes four subsections, referred to as subparts A through D (see http://www.hhs.gov/ohrp/humansubjects/guidance/45cfr46.html). Subpart A specifically lays out the government's policy on protection of human subjects. It addresses the questions of to whom the policy applies; how compliance shall be ascertained; the structure, membership, and mandate of institutional review boards (IRB); and requirements for obtaining and documenting informed consent. Subpart B provides additional protections for pregnant women, fetuses, and newborns; subpart C establishes protections for prisoners; and subpart D addresses the protection of children.

In 1991, 14 additional federal departments and agencies (including the Food and Drug Administration) essentially adopted subpart A of 45CFR46, most often referred to as the "Common Rule," codifying it in their regulations for human subject research. Of note, in July 2011 HHS, along with the Office of Science and Technology Policy, issued an advance notice of proposed rulemaking (ANPR) requesting public comment on how the current regulations for protecting human subjects who participate in research might be modernized and revised (seehttp://www.hhs.gov/ohrp/humansubjects/anprm2011page.html). The rationale for the request to changes in the Common Rule was a need to address changes in research that have occurred since the rules were first promulgated 2–3 decades ago and to ensure that current regulations remained effective and efficient. However, as of December 2013, the Common Rule has not been updated.

Historical and Current Examples of Genetics Research

Genetic research occurs in several discrete areas, each of which raises different ethical concerns. Initially, individuals and families participated in single disease-based studies to try to identify the cause for (typically Mendelian) genetic disorders present in their families. These "family studies" initially used linkage and now use next-generation sequencing technologies of affected individuals, trios, or larger family arrangements to identify the locus of interest. An example would be to assess a family like Amy's to discover highly penetrant dementia genes such as Presenilin 1/2 (*PSEN1* and *PSEN2*) and Amyloid Precursor Protein (*APP*).[15] These situations usually entail a single-use consent process that has the primary purpose of gene/mutation identification for a specific condition present in the family (although some studies allow participants to agree to be recontacted for future participation and/or the use of samples for future studies). Particularly in the early days of clinical genetic testing (before many genetic tests became commercially available), participating in a study like this, even without a promise for family-specific information, was the only way that a family could hope that a predictive genetic test might become available for other family members. Currently most genetic research studies facilitate confirmatory clinical testing through a Clinical Laboratory Improvement Amendement (CLIA) certified laboratory for families with a detectable mutation that is discovered through research testing.

As genetic studies broadened and required much larger sample sizes, genetic biorepositories (sometimes called "bio banks") were established. First started in the early 2000s, these genetic biorepositories were set up to collect large amounts of DNA in conjunction with associated, and often electronic, medical information.[16] Some participants were enrolled as case samples for a specific study purpose but could also serve as "controls" in other studies performed on biorepository samples. Other participants were enrolled more generally, without a specific study purpose in mind. Several US biorepositories are part of a National Human Genome Research Institute (NHGRI) –funded consortium (eMERGE I and II) and have published broadly on their approaches and "lessons learned" from both a logistical and ethical standpoint.[17] A recent survey by Henderson et al. suggests that approximately 79% of biorepositories utilize an "opt in" consent process with 76% using a broad consent approach, 16% allowing limited consent, and 5% allowing both consent approaches.[18,19] The data-storage process for biorepositories varies significantly, but typically entails a de-identification through "hashing" of samples and electronic medical records so that they remain linked and are updated in a longitudinal manner. Some allow for re-identification and/or recontact, while others do not. Biorepository samples and associated data have been used for genome-wide association and other large genetic studies, identifying thousands of genetic loci and typically providing low penetrance risks for common complex disorders of adulthood such as cancers and diabetes. In some cases, biorepository samples undergo whole genome or exome sequencing. Few biorepositories provide aggregate (38%) or individual results (19%) to biorepository participants, however.[18,19]

Finally, as in other areas of medicine, genetic research is also used to document population statistics (e.g., data from newborn screening programs) to clarify the natural history of disorders and as part of clinical trials for treatment of genetic disease. We will not address these areas of research, as they significantly overlap with the ethical issues that arise across all of biomedical research.

Cross-Cutting Ethical Issues in Genetic Research

Several issues span the various types of genetic studies and are of broad relevance, with slightly different impacts depending on the type and process of research in question. These include privacy and data-sharing issues, return of results, commercialization issues and investigator conflicts of interest, multiple use of samples, withdrawal from research, and informed consent. In this section we discuss these cross-cutting ethical issues using examples of how they apply to various types of genetic research studies. All researchers should undergo training in the ethics of human subjects research prior to participation in research teams and should consult their local institutional review boards for guidance as appropriate.

Privacy, Data Sharing, and Interests of Family Members

Privacy and confidentiality are critical in all forms of genetic research, with key issues including potential identifiability and genetic discrimination. Research genomic data and its related phenotypes can cover the full spectrum from "anonymous" (meaning collected without any identifying information) to coded with a clear link to individual information.[20] While people may conceptually understand that full genome sequencing could prove identifiable, recent studies have recently shown that much smaller pieces of genomic data, even from limited SNP data, gene expression data, or microbial DNA (the "microbiome"), make it possible to identify research subjects particularly when combined with other data such as age, zip code, or surname or the use of genealogy databases.[21–30] As such, some authors argue that all genomic research is potentially identifiable and that investigators should be transparent with participants about the mechanisms taken to protect privacy but should not describe studies as "anonymous."[22]

Since 2003, Health Insurance Portability and Accountability Act of 1996 (HIPAA) requirements may include additional notifications and explicit written authorization regarding privacy protections to "individually identifiable health information" or "protected health information (PHI)." PHI is defined by a specific list of items and applies when research is occurring through or using data derived from a "covered entity" defined as an individual health provider, health provider organization (e.g., a practice or hospital), health plan (e.g., a payer), or health information clearinghouse. Currently, waivers to such authorization can be granted through IRBs or privacy boards if they meet specific minimal risk criteria, are used specifically for research preparation only, or include data only from deceased persons, de-identified data, or data from a "limited data set."[31] It is important to note that research performed by an entity not meeting criteria for being a covered entity and that does not use any information or data originating from such is *not* covered by HIPAA. The federal Genetic Information Nondiscrimination Act of 2008 (GINA) and state-based genetic privacy laws may also provide additional protections, primarily around health insurance discrimination and employment discrimination.[32] Rodriguez et al. (2013) provides a good review of policy issues to consider around genomic datasets and attempts to develop federal policies that promote beneficial genomic research while protecting privacy to the greatest extent possible.[33] Finally, the Office of Human Research Protections (OHRP) provides guidance on confidentiality and research data protections,[34] and in 2013 the NIH created a draft Genomic Data Sharing Policy which is expected to be published in final form during 2014.

Genetic studies that utilize linkage or trios to identify a disease-causing gene are typically based on familial comparisons and raise a set of family-specific issues worth consideration. First, such studies can specifically identify mistaken family relationships (e.g., nonpaternity), which is an issue that clinical genetics providers have been familiar with for many years. Separately, family members might be pressured into participating in genetic research studies that may not benefit them in any way. Publication of genetic studies involving rare conditions also raises the issue of identifiability of (and subsequent discrimination against) such families. A case at Virginia Commonwealth University (VCU) in 2000 raised the issue of identifiability of family members identified on published research pedigrees who had not specifically given consent to participate in the research. Bennett provides a good review of the issues that occur around the use of pedigrees in research and publication, providing examples and case studies of ethical issues that arise.[35,36]

Beyond these family-based genetic research studies, recent has trended toward larger datasets (e.g., HapMap, 1000 Genomes, biorepositories), and a genomic or exomic dataset. Additionally, federally funded research typically now requires the deposit of both genotype and phenotypic data into federally based databases such as dbGAP and ClinVar.[37] Data sharing of de-identified genotypes and phenotypic data to approved researchers is meant to facilitate meta-analysis and other "big data" studies. These large datasets are uniquely valuable for data mining, but such broad use—particularly when it may not match the original purpose for which consent was obtained—raises concern for protecting the privacy of research participants. Additionally, many biorepositories allow longitudinal access to electronic medical records, which means that participants may have consented to access at a time before they develop medical conditions that they now wish to maintain as private. The National Institutes of Health provides the option to apply for a certificate of confidentiality, which can provide additional protection such that investigators and their institutions are not compelled to disclose potentially identifying research data in civil, criminal. and administrative settings.[38]

Return of Results

In the early stages of genetic research, few studies returned individual results to participants as research. This was both because such studies were intended to provide generalizable knowledge rather than individual benefit and because the implications of research findings were often poorly understood, with limited clinical validity or utility. Despite this, the return of aggregate research results (e.g., through sharing a publication or describing general findings in a participant newsletter) frequently led to requests for individual research results.[39] As summarized in 2013 by Susan Wolf, many studies addressing participant preferences also suggest that a high percentage (>90%) of research participants desire the return of individual research results.[40] Out of respect for research participants, and given the potential beneficence in returning individual research findings, recent years have seen a transition such that many genetic research studies do provide individual research results related to the primary study purpose, typically after validating the results in a CLIA-approved clinical laboratory. This becomes more challenging when considering research results from biorepositories, where broader consent is obtained and samples may be de-identified before provision to specific researchers making recontact and return of results logistically more complicated and costly. As mentioned earlier, few biorepositories provide aggregate (38%) or individual (19%) results to their participants.[18] Concerns voiced around returning individual research results include the increased financial costs, expertise, and time required of researchers to return such results as well as the conflation of research and clinical care leading to "therapeutic misconception" around the purpose of research participation. Little empiric data addresses the former concern, although the latter is well documented in all areas of medical research. An issue of current controversy is how genomic research studies should consider the potential return of incidental or secondary findings to research participants. An NHGRI workshop was held to consider this issue in February 2014.

Commercialization and Investigator Conflicts of Interest

Intellectual property and patenting are a controversial aspect in the translation from research to clinical genetics practice. In theory patents drive research progress forward by providing incentives to patent holders for public disclosure of their inventions. However, some argue that gene patents decrease access to clinical genetic tests, raise costs, or prevent research and development and improvement of diagnostic services[41,42] The most prominent example, *Association of Molecular Pathology et al. v. Myriad Genetics Inc. et al.*, hereafter referred to as the Myriad case, raised many of these issues and was debated at the Supreme Court level. Sample ownership is another issue that arises as research is translated into clinical care, particularly when partnerships between families and/or advocacy organizations lead to gene discovery and commercial test development and licensure. As an example of positive collaboration, in 2004 the gene for pseudoxanthoma elasticum (PXE) was patented, naming the Executive Director of the PXE Foundation and four scientists on the patent, and all patent rights were given over to the PXE Foundation. In contrast, there was controversy over the 2012 patent of genomic discoveries related to Parkinson disease by the commercial company 23andme and based on participants recruited from a Parkinson disease advocacy group.[43] The relationship between a commercial genetic testing company and research it conducts should be transparent and should follow ethical rules and regulations to ensure that potential conflicts are addressed.[44,45]

Finally since conflicts of interest, specifically financial conflicts, can influence the perception that research design and/or outcomes are biased, the Common Rule and the FDA have disclosure guidelines for potentially serious conflicts. These include but are not limited to compensation, paid consultancies (including legal testimonies and honorarium/speakers fees), equity (including ownership/stock/options), intellectual property (IP) rights (including those on the tested product), and gifts.

Multiple Sample Use and Subjects' Right to Withdraw

Traditionally research samples are used for a single purpose, which is well described to participants as part of the informed consent process. Many studies allow participants to determine whether they wish their samples to be used in other studies or restricted to the single study. In some situations, this requires recontact and reconsent, whereas others are approached more broadly (e.g., the biorepository approach) where participants may not know for what studies their sample is used. Out of respect for participants there should always be a potential to withdraw consent for participation, but particularly in any funded studies where data is deposited into databases such as dbGAP withdrawal may be limited only to future studies and not include removal of a participant's data from prior studies or from deposit into such databases. The Havasupi Indian lawsuit is a very public instance of multiple use of samples that was not previously consented and raises the issue of how this is handled in the consent process.[46] The draft NHGRI genomic data-sharing recommendations propose ways in which this can be handled, including prospective consent in future research, recontact and/or community consultation when possible, and consideration of the spirit of consent for samples where recontact is not possible.

Informed Consent

The process of obtaining informed consent, both for research and clinical practice, is based on the principle of participant's autonomy and, at least in the United States, is governed conceptually by adherence to 45CFR46 and usually reviewed by the center's IRB. In order to consent to participate in research, particularly when given the impression that research is being performed to ascertain specific risks and benefits and that the participant may not directly benefit, it is critical that the participants have the ability to comprehend what is known about the study purpose and potential risks involved.

Informed consent should be seen as a process rather than simply a signature on a consent form, although in practice the consent form is used to outline the key points that should be conveyed to a participant. Key components that should be included are logistics about the study participation (e.g., how long the study will last, the required components to participation), the study purpose, and an outline of the potential benefits and risks (physical, psychosocial, social/legal and financial risks) involved. Typically the focus is on physical risks—the risk of a surgical procedure, a medical treatment, or a blood draw. But in genetic research the emotional and social risks, including loss of privacy and potential discrimination, may be more relevant to decision making than the risk for sample collection through a buccal smear or blood draw. Specifically, decisions related to genetics can be seen as highly personal and with possible psychological impact. Additionally, some genetic research poses a risk for group harms; for example those that examine a specific ethnicity, tribe, or geographic area, such as the Havasupi-related research cited above.[46] In both clinical and research genetic testing, there has consequently been a strong focus on patient/subject autonomy and "informed choice" to promote values-based decision making. Biorepositories and large population studies have also frequently taken a community engagement approach to involve stakeholders and future participants in shaping the approach toward genetic research.[47–51]

Despite this high theoretical standard to promote patient autonomy across all areas of medicine and medical research, actual practice around informed consent varies significantly both between and within study types and institutions. Where risks are high (particularly physical risks), the expectation for comprehension and decision making are held to a higher standard than in situations where there is low risk. A clinical example of this is the comparison between the informed consent approaches for invasive prenatal diagnosis (amniocentesis or CVS) as compared to those for noninvasive screening through maternal serum or ultrasound. There is a moderate amount of research that has studied clinical informed consent processes and found significant variation in clinical practice influenced by time, other clinical setting variables, and provider knowledge and interest. Using time as an example, providers and researchers often have limited time to dedicate to the informed consent process, and patients/subjects may not have the time or "cognitive bandwidth" to process a large amount of complicated information. As a result, patients often have low understanding and recall in both clinical and research settings.[52–54]

With regard specifically to informed consent in genomics research, McGuire and Beskow nicely outline many of the key issues.[55] Informed consent requires participants to comprehend the study purpose and what it will entail, both currently and in the future; genetic and genomic research often involves broad purposes, sometimes not well defined at the time of consent (and often evolving technologically over time). Issues can develop when a new technology or approach is used on stored research samples that may not have been specifically consented for such research. Researchers and their governing IRBs will need to determine whether such additional research is covered by the existing consent, whether recontact and reconsent is required (and even feasible), or if the newly proposed research fits the spirit for which the samples were consented.

Conclusions

Human subjects genetic and genomic research raises a range of ethical issues that vary slightly depending on the specific approach and type of research being performed. Researchers should be cognizant of critical issues at the inception of the study design, including privacy and data-sharing issues, return of results, commercialization issues and investigator conflicts of interest, multiple use of samples, and potential to withdraw from research. Transparency with research participants about the potential risks and benefits of research is a critical and challenging aspect of the informed consent process, particularly in a research area that is rapidly evolving.

BOX 8.1 Nuremberg Code

The voluntary consent of the human subject is absolutely essential.

The experiment should be such as to yield fruitful results for the good of society, unprocurable by other methods or means of study, and not random and unnecessary in nature.

The experiment should be so designed and based on the results of animal experimentations and knowledge of the natural history of the disease or other problem under study that the anticipated results will justify the performance of the experiment.

The experiment should be conducted as to avoid all unnecessary physical and mental suffering and injury.

No experiment should be conducted where there is a priori reason to believe that death or disabling injury will occur; except, perhaps, in those experiments where the experimental physicians also serve as subjects.

The degree of risk to be taken should never exceed that determined by the humanitarian importance of the problem to be solved by the experiment.

Proper preparations should be made and adequate facilities provided to protect the experimental subject against even remove possibilities of injury, disability, or death.

Only scientifically qualified persons should conduct the experiment. The highest degree of skill and care should be required through all stages of the experiment of those who conduct or engage in the experiment.

During the course of the experiment, the human subject should be at liberty to bring the experiment to an end if he has reached the physical or mental state where continuation of the experiment seems to him to be impossible.

During the course of the experiment, the scientist in charge must be prepared to terminate the experiment at any stage, if he has probably [sic] cause to believe, in the exercise of the good faith, superior skill and careful judgment required of him that a continuation of the experiment is likely to result in injury, disability, or death to the experimental subject.

Source: Trials of War Criminals before the Nuremberg Military Tribunals under Control Council Law No. 10. Washington, D.C.: U.S. Government Printing Office. 1949. pp. 181–182.

REFERENCES

1. Trials of War Criminals before the Nuremberg Military Tribunals under Control Council Law No. 10. Washington, DC: U.S. Government Printing Office. 1949. pp. 181–182.
2. Weindling, P. (2001). The origins of informed consent: the International Scientific Commission on Medical War Crimes, and the Nuremburg code. *Bulletin of the History of Medicine.* 75(1):37–71.
3. Ghooi, R.B. (2011). The Nuremberg Code–a critique. *Perspectives in Clinical Research.* 2(2):72–76.
4. Markman, J.R., Markman, M. (2007). Running an ethical trial 60 years after the Nuremberg Code. *The Lancet Oncology.* 8(12):1139–1146.
5. The World Medical Association Declaration of Helsinki: Ethical principles for medical research involving human subjects. (2013). *Journal of the American Medical Association.* 310(20):2191–2194.
6. The World Medical Association Declaration on Ethical Considerations Regarding Health Databases (2001). Available from: http://www.rewi.uni-jena.de/rewimedia/Downloads/LS_Ruffert/Ethical_Codes/WMA_Declaration+on+Ethical+Considerations+regarding+Health+Databases.pdf.
7. Organization for Economic Co-Operation and Development (OECD). (2009). OECD Guidelines on Human Biobanks and Genetic Research Databases Available from: http://www.oecd.org/sti/biotech/44054609.pdf.
8. Genomics and World Health: Report of the Advisory Committee on Health Research, 2002.
9. United Nations Educational Scientific and Cultural Organization. (1997). Universal declaration on the human genome and human rights (revised draft). *Bulletin of Medical Ethics.* 126:9–11.
10. United Nations Educational Scientific and Cultural Organization. (2003). International Declaration on Human Genetic Data (2003). Available from: http://portal.unesco.org/en/ev.php-URL_ID=17720&URL_DO=DO_TOPIC&URL_SECTION=201.html.
11. Beauchamp, T.L., Saghai, Y. (2012). The historical foundations of the research-practice distinction in bioethics. *Theoretical Medicine and Bioethics.* 33(1):45–56.

12. National Commission for the Protection of Human Subjects of Biomedical and Behavioral Reserach. (1979). The Belmont Report: Ethical principles and guidelines for the protection of human subjects of research. Available from: http://www.hhs.gov/ohrp/humansubjects/guidance/belmont.html.
13. Nijhawan, L.P., Janodia, M.D., Muddukrishna, B.S., Bhat, K.M., Bairy, K.L., Udupa, N., et al. (2013). Informed consent: issues and challenges. *Journal of Advanced Pharmaceutical Technology & Research*. 4(3):134–140.
14. Sims, J.M. (2010). A brief review of the Belmont Report. *Dimensions of Critical Care Nursing*. 29(4):173–174.
15. Rogaev, E.I., Sherrington, R., Rogaeva, E.A., Levesque, G., Ikeda, M., Liang, Y., et al. (1995). Familial Alzheimer's disease in kindreds with missense mutations in a gene on chromosome 1 related to the Alzheimer's disease type 3 gene. *Nature*. 376(6543):775–778.
16. Austin, M.A., Harding, S., McElroy, C. (2003). Genebanks: a comparison of eight proposed international genetic databases. *Community Genetics*. 6(1):37–45.
17. Gottesman, O., Kuivaniemi, H., Tromp, G., Faucett, W.A., Li, R., Manolio, T.A., et al. (2013). The Electronic Medical Records and Genomics (eMERGE) Network: past, present, and future. *Genetics in Medicine*.15(10):761–771.
18. Henderson, G.E., Cadigan, R.J., Edwards, T.P., Conlon, I., Nelson, A.G., Evans, J.P., et al. (2013). Characterizing biobank organizations in the U.S.: results from a national survey. *Genome Medicine*. 5(1):3.
19. Henderson, G.E., Edwards, T.P., Cadigan, R.J., Davis, A.M., Zimmer, C., Conlon, I., et al. (2013). Stewardship practices of U.S. biobanks. *Science Translational Medicine*. 5(215):215cm7.
20. Lowrance, W.W., Collins, F.S. (2007). Ethics. Identifiability in genomic research. *Science*. 317(5838):600–602.
21. Bohannon, J. (2013). Genetics. Genealogy databases enable naming of anonymous DNA donors. *Science*. 339(6117):262.
22. Schmidt, H., Callier, S. (2012). How anonymous is "anonymous?" Some suggestions towards a coherent universal coding system for genetic samples. *Journal of Medical Ethics*. 38(5):304–309.
23. Malin, B., Sweeney, L. (2001). Re-identification of DNA through an automated linkage process. *Proceedings /AMIA Annual Symposium*. 423–427.

24. Schadt, E.E. (2012). The changing privacy landscape in the era of big data. *Molecular Systems Biology*. 8:612.
25. Schadt, E.E., Woo, S., Hao, K. (2012). Bayesian method to predict individual SNP genotypes from gene expression data. *Nature Genetics*. 44(5):603–608.
26. Gymrek, M., McGuire, A.L., Golan, D., Halperin, E., Erlich, Y. (2013). Identifying personal genomes by surname inference. *Science*. 339(6117):321–324.
27. Malin, B.A., Sweeney, L.A. (2002). Inferring genotype from clinical phenotype through a knowledge based algorithm. *Pacific Symposium on Biocomputing Pacific Symposium on Biocomputing*. 41–52.
28. Im, H.K., Gamazon, E.R., Nicolae, D.L., Cox, N.J. (2012). On sharing quantitative trait GWAS results in an era of multiple-omics data and the limits of genomic privacy. *American Journal of Human Genetics*. 90(4):591–598.
29. Schloissnig, S., Arumugam, M., Sunagawa, S., Mitreva, M., Tap, J., Zhu, A., et al. (2013). Genomic variation landscape of the human gut microbiome. *Nature*. 493(7430):45–50.
30. Lin, Z., Owen, A.B., Altman, R.B. (2004). Genetics. Genomic research and human subject privacy. *Science*. 305(5681):183.
31. US Department of Health and Human Services (USDoHHS). Health Information Privacy 2003. Available from: http://www.hhs.gov/ocr/privacy/hipaa/understanding/coveredentities/research.html.
32. Genetic Information Nondscrimination Act of 2008. Pub.L. 110–233, 122 Stat. 881, enacted May 21, 2008.
33. Rodriguez, L.L., Brooks, L.D., Greenberg, J.H., Green, E.D (2013). Research ethics. The complexities of genomic identifiability. *Science*. 339(6117):275–276.
34. National Institutes of Health (2003). Final NIH Statement on Sharing Research Data. http://grants.nih.gov/grants/guide/notice-files/NOT-OD-03-032.html
35. Bennett, R.L., French, K.S., Resta, R.G., Doyle, D.L. (2008). Standardized human pedigree nomenclature: update and assessment of the recommendations of the National Society of Genetic Counselors. *Journal of Genetic Counseling*. 17(5):424–433.
36. Steinhaus, K.A., Bennett, R.L., Resta, R.G., Uhrich, S.B., Doyle, D.L., Markel, D.S., et al. (1995). Inconsistencies in pedigree

symbols in human genetics publications: a need for standardization. *American Journal of Medical Genetics*. 56(3):291–295.

37. NCBI. What is ClinVar? AccessedFebruary 24, 2014. Available from: http://www.ncbi.nlm.nih.gov/clinvar/intro.
38. National Institutes of Health. Certificates of Confidentiality Kiosk. (2002). Accessed February 19, 2014. Available from: http://grants.nih.gov/grants/policy/coc.
39. Beskow, L.M., Burke, W. (2010). Offering individual genetic research results: context matters. *Science Translational Medicine*. 2(38):38cm20.
40. Wolf, S.M. (2013). Return of individual research results and incidental findings: facing the challenges of translational science. *Annual Review of Genomics and Human Genetics*. 14:557–577.
41. Cho, M.K., Illangasekare, S., Weaver, M.A., Leonard, D.G., Merz, J.F. (2003). Effects of patents and licenses on the provision of clinical genetic testing services. *The Journal of Molecular Diagnostics*. 5(1):3–8.
42. Ormond, K.E., Cho, M. (2014). Translating personalized medicine using new genetic technologies in clinical practice: the ethical issues. *Personalized Medicine*. 11(2):211–222.
43. Wojcicki, A. (2012). Announcing 23andMe's first patent. Accessed February 24, 2014. Available from: http://blog.23andme.com/news/announcements/announcing-23andmes-first-patent/.
44. Sterckx, S., Cockbain, J., Howard, H., Huys, I., Borry, P. (2013). "Trust is not something you can reclaim easily:" patenting in the field of direct-to-consumer genetic testing. *Genetics in Medicine*. 15(5):382–387.
45. Tobin, S.L., Cho, M.K., Lee, S.S., Magnus, D.C., Allyse, M., Ormond, K.E., et al. (2012). Customers or research participants? Guidance for research practices in commercialization of personal genomics. *Genetics in Medicine*. 14(10):833–835.
46. Garrison, N.A., Cho, M.K. (2013). Awareness and acceptable practices: IRB and researcher reflections on the Havasupai lawsuit. *AJOB Primary Research*. 4(4):55–63.
47. Haldeman, K.M., Cadigan, R.J., Davis, A., Goldenberg, A., Henderson, G.E., Lassiter, D., et al. (2014). Community engagement in US biobanking: multiplicity of meaning and method. *Public Health Genomics*. 17(2):84–94.

48. Godard, B., Ozdemir, V., Fortin, M., Egalite, N. (2010). Ethnocultural community leaders' views and perceptions on biobanks and population specific genomic research: a qualitative research study. *Public Understanding of Science*. 19(4): 469–485.
49. Hartzler, A., McCarty, C.A., Rasmussen, L.V., Williams, M.S., Brilliant, M., Bowton, E.A., et al. (2013). Stakeholder engagement: a key component of integrating genomic information into electronic health records. *Genetics in Medicine*. 15(10):792–801.
50. Lemke, A.A., Wu, J.T., Waudby, C., Pulley, J., Somkin, C.P., Trinidad, S.B. (2010). Community engagement in biobanking: Experiences from the eMERGE Network. *Genomics, Society, and Policy / ESRC Genomics Network*. 6(3):35–52.
51. O'Doherty, K.C., Burgess, M.M. (2009). Engaging the public on biobanks: outcomes of the BC biobank deliberation. *Public Health Genomics*. 12(4):203–215.
52. Cassileth, B.R., Zupkis, R.V., Sutton-Smith, K., March, V. (1980). Informed consent—why are its goals imperfectly realized? *The New England Journal of Medicine*. 302(16):896–900.
53. Mason, S.A., Allmark, P.J. (2000). Obtaining informed consent to neonatal randomised controlled trials: interviews with parents and clinicians in the Euricon study. *Lancet*. 356(9247):2045–2051.
54. Kusec, S., Oreskovic, S., Skegro, M., Korolija, D., Busic, Z., Horzic, M. (2006). Improving comprehension of informed consent. *Patient Education and Counseling*. 60(3):294–300.
55. McGuire, A.L., Beskow, L.M. (2010). Informed consent in genomics and genetic research. *Annual Review of Genomics and Human Genetics*. 11:361–381.

Index

b denotes box; *f* denotes figure; *t* denotes table

www.ingramcontent.com/pod-product-compliance
Ingram Content Group UK Ltd.
Pitfield, Milton Keynes, MK11 3LW, UK
UKHW041353190726
13851UKWH00014B/92